# Anti Inflammatory Diet

Guide + Cookbook: cleanse your body in an healthy and easy way, reduce inflammation naturally with the Alkaline Diet.
(Bonus Recipes and Meal Preps Included)

Mark J. Patterson

# Table of contents

# Introduction

Thank you for downloading a copy of this book! I am sure you are as excited as I am to start your weight loss journey by switching your diet to alkaline. This book will educate you on the benefits and basics of the alkaline diet as well as go over how to cleanse your body of unwanted toxins. In addition, it also covers a wide range of various types of herbal medicine and the benefits of using them.

Flip through to discover a plethora of different ways to eat alkaline without sacrificing the fun of food! Easy to intermediate recipes for breakfast, lunch, dinner, dessert, and snacks are included for you to master. These recipes keep in mind that it is hard to maintain a healthy diet with a busy schedule, so these confections are great to make ahead or on a whim.

Cooking experience is not needed to try these recipes! Most recipes just require basic cooking materials like baking sheets and pans for low-stress cooking that doesn't require you to go out and wreck your wallet. Each recipe will provide the amount of time it takes, the yielded servings, the difficulty level, an ingredients list, and detailed steps to make preparation a breeze.

This book is filled with useful information to guide you on your first steps towards healthy living. With so many diet and health books out there, thank you for choosing this one! Happy cooking!

# Basics of an Alkaline Diet

In a world of fast, faster, and fastest, it is easy to become tied up and overlook your most important possession: your body. When it comes to a compromise between a busy schedule and a healthy body, the latter usually slides into the shadows. The hardest part of diets is that they are difficult to maintain and easy to ignore, and we have a tendency to put it off until it is too late. "I'll go to the gym starting next week." "Oh well I had a cookie today so I might as well start tomorrow." "But I have a cook-out party coming up this weekend so maybe I'll just wait until next week to start." The excuses are never-ending, especially if the diet plan is hard to incorporate into normal day to day life. Enter the Alkaline Diet! Give yourself the gift of a healthy body and your life will transform. All it takes is deciding to take the first step.

## What is it?

If you're looking for an easy way to be healthy and lose some lbs., the alkaline diet is for you. The alkaline diet is a weight loss solution that is based on monitoring your body's pH. The term pH refers to "potential of hydrogen" and measure the acidity and alkalinity of any substance. The scale stretches from 0-14 with zero being extremely acidic and fourteen being extremely alkaline. Neutral pH is usually considered to be 7, but our bodies are set at a slightly alkaline pH of 7.4. The difference may seem small but our bodies work hard to maintain this level because even the smallest of rising or falling in pH level can cause serious health problems.

 At first glance, this might seem complicated and difficult to maintain, but it is actually a great and easy way to start a journey to healthy living. This diet focuses on the foods you eat and the residue they leave in your body. It targets specific health issues like weight loss, bone health, and proper sleep.

## pH Levels

The main most important goal of the entire alkaline diet focuses on changing your body's pH level. Once this is achieved, you can fully reap the beneficial value. How exactly is this done, and how is it measured?

Potential hydrogen is what pH stands for. When deciding pH levels, hydrogen ions, and hydroxide ions become significantly important. When adding water to an acid or base, hydroxide ions or hydrogen ions are produced. This is how we will determine whether or not this is an acid or a base substance.

One common acid is known as hydrochloric acid. When added to water, it will produce hydrogen ions. We cannot see this with the human eye, but with scientific methods, it will be revealed. The abundance of hydrogen ions over hydroxide ions is what makes this an acid. As hydrogen ions are increasing, the more acidic a substance is. The highest pH level of acidity would be one.

Alkaline substances can also be labeled as bases. When added to water, they produce hydroxide ions in abundance rather than hydrogen ions. With more hydroxide ions than hydrogen ions, the substance is more alkaline. For example, a substance with a pH value of twelve is more alkaline than a substance with a pH of eight.

There is one other category besides the ones previously discussed, acid or base (alkaline.) This is a substance that falls under the exact pH value of seven. This is what it is called neutral. One main substance that falls under the value of seven is one we all know well. Pure water. Hardly any other substances are known to have an exact pH of seven. Often times, substances will have a pH of seven followed by a small decimal amount. This makes them alkaline instead of neutral.

Now, with an understanding of the pH scale, another method will be introduced. Food substances can be applied to this pH scale. They have predetermined levels of acidity or alkalinity. However, their method of determining pH is quite different. Metabolism is a process where the body breaks down food to gain energy. This is also called catabolism. The body does this to supply nutrients it cannot create itself. Manmade attempts to recreate this consist of burning food to produce ash. Then, the ash is tested to discover the pH of the food. This process, which was titled 'ash analysis,' was found to be quite inaccurate.

Currently, a different formula is used. The two results that can come from this test is positive and negative. Positive would mean that once the food has reached the kidneys, after being metabolized, it remains very acidic. Alkaline foods, however, would be labeled as a negative score. This formula is called potential renal acid load. Renal would be describing the kidneys.

The alkaline diet takes alkaline foods to balance the body's pH. It creates an alkaline ash leftover from metabolism as previously discussed. Common household food items support acidic properties to develop in the body. The kidney performs a task that eliminates acids from our body daily. However, it is limited in the amount it can eliminate per day. Any acid that can no longer be eliminated is stored within the body. This excess acid is what this diet aspires to eliminate. There is no possibility of this happening because of the method imposed by the diet. Alkaline foods will result in alkaline ash. In addition, this keeps unneeded, unhealthy acidic waste from your body.

Cheese has a pH level of 5. Because of this, it is considered an acid. As you go through the steps of this diet, the cheese will be prohibited. However, there are still foods higher in acidity to be wary of. Stronger acids are closer to one. Food-wise this would be substances like alcohol or even eggs.

Coffee is one common household drink that is also high in acidity. Its energizing effects are sure to be loved by the forced early risers, but its four-point five pH level isn't exactly healthy for everyday consumption. This option isn't exactly body pH friendly for our diet. The alkaline smoothies themselves can be a great replacement.

This being said, a confusing topic for most beginners may be the amount of fruit that is included in this diet. If the fruit has such a low pH, shouldn't it be ruled out? This is, in fact, false for a very good reason. It's originally low pH before consumption is converted to more alkaline ash as it reaches the kidneys. This gives it a low potential renal acid load score. As a result, it is alkalizing to the body. Fruit makes up a large part of this diet for this reason.

The most common foods you must now stay away from are most meats. Chicken, beef, tuna, pork, and others are among these. Dairy products must also be limited for its acidity. Alcohol of any type and microwavable dinners are to be strayed away from for the same reasons. If in doubt of an item's pH levels, it can always be searched for.

## The Dangers of Excess Acid

A common misconception is that an alkaline diet works to change your body's pH. This is not true. The human body is hardwired to maintain a pH somewhere around 7.35, slightly alkaline. Excess acid usually a result of one of the following. The first is the dietary choices. When you consume a large number of processed sugars and fats and your body metabolizes them, those food turn into acid. In addition, the Western diet circulates around acid-heavy foods like meat and carbs which makes it easy to get a buildup of acid in your body. When you consume a large amount of these foods, the body attempts to maintain its pH balance. In order to combat excess acid, your body reacts in a multitude of ways that long-term can have a negative effect on bodily health. To restore its pH back to the proper balance, the body pulls alkaline buffers from all over. Extra cholesterol is created to neutralize the extra acid which is why so many western-diet eating people have high cholesterol. Your body pulls iron from red blood cells which can lead to anemia, while potassium is stolen from your muscles, deteriorating them. The most dangerous effect is when your body begins to pull calcium from your bones. Over a period of time, this can weaken bone health and eventually lead to osteoporosis.

Another cause of high body acidity has to do with the environment you are exposed to. When the body is exposed to infection, pollution, and other toxins long term, it begins to burden the immune system. Your body fires up to help out the immune system and when your reserves eventually run out, your body enters a state of distress that results in the build-up of acid.

Excess acid is also a stressor on your body that can lead to inflammation and poor cell health. Acidic foods work to decrease your energy by affecting your muscles efficiency. When your muscles become inflamed, they tighten and have a much harder time expanding and contracting. That means you have to work harder every time you move. Switching over to an alkaline diet will give you extra energy to combat your busy schedule while promoting healthy cell generation to keep you in tip-top shape.

## Warning Signs

Acidic diets often are found to be the comfort food of most people. Why should you stray away from this, and how does continuing these habits hurt you? To begin with, it's drastically unhealthy. Further down the road, medical complications may occur. Negative effects can appear in many forms. One of these is the process of gaining weight. If your diet is heavily contrasting efforts to lose weight, you will never get anywhere. Exercise and drinking water can't reverse the effects of a bad diet.

Acid reflux is another negative of unhealthy eating. Often symptoms of this include burning pain, bloating, excessive burping, or even blood in your vomit or stools. When food enters the stomach through a small valve, similar to a small flap, it is deposited into the stomach. The flap normally functions as a one-way system. The stomach breaks this food apart with its very potent acid. The stomach lining itself is meant to protect the organ from its acid. However, unhealthy diets cause this entire system to malfunction. The stomach's contents, acids, and foods alike are expelled back through the valve from which it came. This causes a burning sensation most call heartburn.

Gradual tooth decay may even result from the daily or overconsumption of energy drinks, acidic juices, and sugary sodas. Skin problems, bone loss, fatigue, and kidney stones are all bad things to come of having such a highly acidic diet. A great amount of pain can be caused by bad choices. Your body will thank you should you commit to the alkaline diet. Those who have preexisting conditions resulting from highly acidic diets should heavily consider making the change. Not only will this ease your symptoms, but you'll be able to eliminate the problem at its source.

## The Benefits of Alkaline

Along with keeping your body functioning at a neutral stable level, adding extra alkaline has loads of other preventative health benefits. Studies have shown that cancer cells tend to thrive in acidic environments. Cutting down on acidic foods and starting an alkaline heavy diet can be a quick and easy step to prevent cancer in the future. Because it is plant-based, the alkaline diet is also beneficial to lowering the risk of heart disease, and kidney disease. If you are a sufferer of chronic kidney stones or kidney infections, this diet is a great choice for you!

The most effectively proven result of the alkaline diet, however, is weight loss. Scientists are still in debate over the specific causation of alkaline eating in regards to cancer and heart disease, but one proven effect of this diet is weight loss. The requirements of this diet (that we will go over later) steer clear of foods high in fats and sugars and pushes the consumption of fresh fruits and vegetables. Cutting unhealthy fats and sugars, as well as processed foods, out of your diet will promote healthy weight loss that doesn't depend on fasting, counting calories, or working out.

The food this diet requires is healthy. Vegetables, fruits, nuts, and others contribute to altering the body's pH levels. The diet tends to be lower in calories for the eater. This process isn't majorly targeted for weight loss, but the body will most likely be the subject of weight loss. Maintaining your weight will become increasingly easier as you progress with this diet. Although this benefit is sure to have a positive impact, other benefits are what makes the alkaline diet so desirable. Conditions very prominent in major areas can be easily avoided by making the right food choices. Risk factors are easily pushed away from mind when this ideal diet is put to the test. It brings to mind the question of 'why not start now?'

The general term 'heart disease' affects a big portion of today's population. The chart above demonstrates the percentage of the population affected by heart disease. In addition, it relays the gender difference of each major age group. Most of these may lead to multiple health complications or even death. One of the more common conditions labeled as heart disease is known as coronary heart disease. Plaque buildup in the arteries, the cause of coronary heart disease, can often lead to heart failure. The plaque itself is caused by frequent poor diet choices. The foods which cause this tend to be more acidic. Cheese, butter, and processed meats are some of the acidic choices that cause plaque buildup. Poor diet, lack of exercise, obesity, and overuse of alcohol are some common risk factors to the conditions which fall under heart disease, such as this one. The alkaline diet eliminates these risk factors with its food restriction principles. The change from acidic to alkaline foods can prevent or even improve the negative effects of heart disease.

In addition, diabetes develops from unhealthy lifestyle choices. The foods people consume are often bad for the body and it takes a toll on the body. Often, this can lead to devastating effects. Excessive or increased thirst, sluggishness, and blurry vision are some of the symptom's patients suffer through. Even more so, diabetes itself can increase your risk of deadlier diseases. Diabetes can even cause damage to the body's organs. One of the organs which might be affected is the kidney.

A chronic kidney disorder is just one of the many conditions that can result from having diabetes. Progression of this disease may even result in kidney failure. The disease itself causes kidney function to drastically increase, so it may not be able to regulate pH levels as it usually does. Another condition related to the kidneys is known as kidney stones. Uric acid stones may form from overconsumption of acidic proteins resulting in pain and even urine complications. This is where the alkaline diet becomes readily helpful. It's the principle of lowering pH levels is proven to improve the outcomes of having chronic kidney disorders. The diet may even lower health costs as the body is improving. Concerning kidney stones, the alkaline diet will prohibit the formation of this with its food plan.

Chronic acidosis is yet another illness where excess amounts of acidic substances in the body can cause harm. This condition can lead to inflammation, headaches, back pain, and more. Following these meal plans can result in the lessening or even eventual, complete termination of these symptoms.

All these diseases and more can easily be avoided or helped in some way. The most surprising condition which can be helped is still yet to be discussed. Cancer is a deadly disease that most people worry about. Sadly, there is no cure, but it can be prevented. The alkaline diet is a shining

beacon in this dreadful prospect. Read further to find out
why this can be.

Highly acidic foods lower our bodies pH and leave us open
to health risks. One of these is the very deadly disease
known as cancer. If we were to absolve the negative food
choices we make, then the number of health conditions we
put ourselves at risk for would lower.

Cancer cells tend to flourish much more quickly in acidic
environments. As there is very often causes of cancer being
found in late stages, everyone should offer much attention
to pushing away any risk factor possible. Genetics is not
something we can change, but our life choices are in our
hands to decide. The first step we can take is what we put
into our bodies.

This is where all components of the diet come into play.
The pH of your body is altered by all that is consumed. As
discussed partially earlier, it has to do with leftover ash
product after food is used for energy. Your diet, having
been changed, is now resulting in your body pH is more
alkaline. It is healthier to be this way. Foods regularly

consumed are energy inducing and body positive. Should the ash still be considered more acidic in nature, cancer cells are more likely to develop.

The alkaline diet severely cuts back on eating any kind of processed meats. This turns out to be amazingly beneficial to any alkaline dieter. Why? There is a known link connecting these foods to developing cancer. When cooking meat at high temperatures, it becomes very carcinogenic. This means the body is at an increased risk for cancer by consuming these because of what it produces under these conditions. The heat that is producing harmful byproducts is what makes this so.

Eggs, which are prohibited from this diet, are known to increase the risk of prostate cancer. With eliminating this from your diet, the established health risk lowers. Cholesterol, in high levels, are what causes them to be so warned against. In addition, its high acidity level already puts it off of the diet itself.

These foods are stricken from this diet and rightfully so. For those who suffer from cancer, the alkaline diet is not meant to serve as a replacement for medical treatment. However, switching your diet to purely alkaline foods may allow you to become healthier. A healthier body is more able to survive and stand the extensive treatments cancer patients must go through. Switching your diet may even be recommended by a nutritionist. With the energy and now more alkaline body pH, survival rates can increase.

## Alkaline Diet Guidelines

Now for the important part: what can you eat? Just because something *tastes* acidic, doesn't mean that it will have an acidic effect on your body. For example, when lemons are digested they are actually highly alkaline while milk, when digested, is highly acidic. There are of course food restrictions on this diet, but don't get nervous yet. The alkaline diet promotes choosing from a much wider range of food than the usual Western diet normally contains. This means a larger variety of healthy nutrients for your body to use. It also means more fun with food and space for you to experiment with a multitude of dishes. Try to base your food intake on the list below.

High alkalizing:

- Greens (avocadoes, kale, and other dark greens are the best)
- Garlic
- Fennel
- Sea vegetables
- Sweet potatoes
- Sprouted seeds and grains
- Non-dairy milk
- Tomatoes
- Lemons
- Sea salt
- Raw almonds
- Fresh herbs
- Stevia
- Cold-pressed oils
- Tofu

Neutral:

- Raw honey
- Lentils
- Nut cheeses
- Cacao

- Water

Neutral/Acidic:

- Agave
- Brown rice syrup
- Dates
- Wild salmon
- Oysters

Acidic:

- Red meat
- Chicken
- Pork
- Shrimp
- Turkey
- Peanuts
- Pasta
- Eggs
- Bread
- White rice

Highly Acidic

- Alcohol

- Milk
- Ice cream
- Artificial sweeteners
- Margarine
- Chocolate
- Jelly
- Coffee
- Non-herbal tea
- Fried foods
- Processed foods
- Candy
- Soda

Eating alkaline revolves mainly around fresh fruits and vegetables. Basically, the rule of thumb is the greener it is the more alkaline it is. (So if you slip up to get the spinach ready!) Steer clear of foods high in sugar and fats, especially processed foods. These are never a good idea, regardless of the diet, you are following. Processed foods in abundance only work to fill the body with toxins and clog the way for helpful nutrients.

Though fruit is a suggested food for this diet, it still is a sugar-heavy food and should be considered a treat for the day. Fruits toe the line between fresh and healthy and high in sugar. While a few pieces a day are a great addition, too many can cause a spike in sugar, reversing the health effects. Stick to just a handful a day for a balanced diet.

As far as protein goes, try to steer towards plant-based proteins like tofu and beans. However, protein is very important to a healthy body so if you are going to cheat somewhere, this would be the place. The recipes that are included in this book are based on a full alkaline nutritional plan, but topping a bowl with a lightly seasoned chicken breast or a hardboiled egg won't make or break this diet. Experts say that people should try to stick to the 80/20 rule. Try to make 80% of your food intake alkaline for a healthy body and mind.

Dairy should be avoided as it is very high in fat and acid. Luckily, it is easy to substitute milk and cheese with non-dairy products like almond and coconut milk. Nut cheeses are also a great substitute to add a bit of extra flavor on top of a salad or pizza. With these recipes, you'll hardly taste the difference, but you will for sure feel a difference as you transition into this healthy living style.

The hardest part of this diet for a lot of people is the fact that it cuts out caffeinated beverages and alcohol. Coffee, to the dismay of many, is also on the list of things you should avoid. If you're a coffee addict, try switching over to green tea which has a pretty neutral pH. Sodas and sugary cocktail drinks have zero health benefits and should be avoided at all costs. Not only are they packed with sugar, but they also contain a plethora of chemicals that bog down the body. To commit to a naturally healthy lifestyle, these beverages should be cut out.  For alcohol, unfortunately, there are no quick and easy substitutes. Try to avoid alcoholic beverages to the best of your ability. However, with all of these restrictions, it is important to remember that a diet shouldn't mean putting your life on hold and enjoying yourself isn't a crime. Healthy living is all about balance so if you slip up or cheat on your diet, do not beat yourself up! Just focus on increasing your intake of alkaline foods to set your body's balance back to neutral.

## Alkaline Boosters

A great thing to have on hand during the alkaline diet plan is supplements. They come in many forms for you to choose your favorite, and they all help to keep your body's alkaline intake on track. One option is pH drops. Tap water is generally acidic, so to give your diet a boost or to catch up on the days that you go acid-overboard, add a couple of drops to give your water an alkalizing effect. Another popular option is alkaline salts. These are primarily calcium, potassium, magnesium, and sodium. A great addition to any healthy lifestyle is omega oils. These oils, such as omega 3, omega 6, omega 9, and coconut oil, keep your body full of important nutrients.

All of these tips don't matter without hydration. Hydration is at the core of a healthy body, and the health benefits of this diet plan are useless without it. That's why it's important to drink, drink, and drink more! The average person should be drinking at least 7 oz. of water for every 10 lbs. of body weight in order to maintain proper body functions. If you're drinking less than that daily, then your body is most likely not functioning at its best. Water also flushes out harmful toxins and prepares the body for nutrients. Paired with the alkaline diet plan, proper hydration leads to the full absorption of nutrients effectively increasing the diet's results.

Having the correct amount of hydration in a day also contributes to the weight loss effect of this diet by curbing your appetite. When our bodies call for food or water, sometimes it is hard to distinguish between the two. Often enough, the feeling we mistake for hunger is actually thirsting. Proper hydration not only keeps the body functioning properly, but it also ensures that you aren't just eating because you are bored.

It is important to note, however, that for alkalizing effects, you should be drinking pure water, not tap water. Tap water is usually acidic in nature, so you'll want to avoid it as much as possible. An easy solution for this is to buy a filtered water pitcher. It will make sure you always have pure water on hand without harming the environment with excessive plastic bottles. (Because to live natural and healthy we should make sure the earth is healthy too!)

# Alkaline Diet as a Weight Loss Tool

There are many different ways to utilize the alkaline diet depending on what results you are looking for, but if you want to shed a few lbs., eating alkaline is worth considering. The build-up of weight can be a result of eating too much acidic food. It is one of the body's defense mechanisms. To combat excess acid, the body will sometimes store it in fatty tissue. The more acid that floods the body from then on will result in an increase in fat.

Start at step one of conquering weight loss with an alkaline cleanse (check out the cleanse chapter that follows). Weight loss efforts are most effective when starting from scratch. Toxins and other residue hanging around can inhibit your efforts. As this book is all about easy, affordable, and manageable healthy living, the cleanse is included so you can see the fastest results. This diet plan is the real deal. There are no instant "fat-melting" solutions here, only usable tips for a healthy living style. Healthy living is a choice to work for a better style of living. It will not come easy, but these are tools to help you on this journey.

The recipes included in this book are full of toxin-clearers and nutrient-boosters that will keep your metabolism chugging along. The alkaline diet is such a great tool for weight loss because it cuts out all the foods that lead to fat build-ups, such as processed sugars and fats. These are replaced with nutrient-filled fresh foods to boost your energy. This energy can then be used towards exercise to increase the rate of weight loss.

This diet is perfect for those trying to lose weight in a healthy way because it doesn't depend on calorie restriction. You do not have to deprive your body of food, nor do you have to sit through stomach grumbling temper tantrums. This diet is unique in that it encourages you to eat healthy delicious foods that you actually want to eat.

# Cleanse Your Body

Everything we eat leaves a residue behind, similar to ash. Your insides get coated with it every time you ingest food. If you have spent a long period of time with an acid-heavy diet, it would be worth your while to do a 7-day alkaline cleanse to start with a clean slate. Wipe your insides clear of harmful toxins and start on your path to healthy living!

## What is it?

A cleanse is a bit different than a diet plan in that it is extremely restricted and a short-term plan. The idea is to restrict your intake of certain foods for a short period of time to get a fresh foundation for your diet. An alkaline cleanse is no different. You'll want to stick to raw fruits and vegetables, tofu, and certain nuts while steering clear of processed sugars and fats. This will clear your digestive tract of harmful toxins so you'll be able to absorb the full effect of the nutrients you are consuming.

# Why does it?

Cleansing your body is especially important if you have been off and on other diets in the past. Just because you are dieting, does not mean your body is in a healthy state. A lot of diets increase acidity levels to a skyrocketing level while requiring you to starve yourself. This causes the body to go into a dangerous state of distress that we learned causes acid to be released in abundance. To get the full impact of this diet, a cleanse is the best place to start.

Some of the best alkaline foods to ingest are:

- Beets
- Broccoli
- Avocado
- Spinach
- Kiwi
- Olive oil
- Tofu
- Almonds
- Ginger
- Cinnamon

- Apples
- Kale
- Onions
- Peppers

Some foods to avoid at all costs during your cleanse are:

- Cheese
- Coffee
- Yogurt
- Sugar
- Processed foods
- Bread
- Alcohol
- Meats

Remember, this high restriction only needs to last as long as you desire your cleanse to be. Experts recommend performing a cleanse for 3 to 10 days to give your system adequate time to clear out. It's also important to note that restriction does not refer to the amount of food taken in but rather the type of food taken in. This diet does not require you to fast or go hungry, which is why it is so great for healthy weight loss. If you're not big on snacking on raw veggies, flip through this book to the drinks and smoothies recipe section. There are some great recipes using raw fruits and vegetables and other alkaline high ingredients that are perfect for a cleanse. Try a variety of flavors or have fun trying your own hand at mixing recipes. it is quick, easy, and makes cleaning fun! Because healthy living shouldn't have to be torture.

That's why this book is here; to provide you with numerous ways to make a healthy diet delicious and easy. When you think of a cleanse, do not imagine yourself drinking watery kale juice or miserably munching on celery. Picture yourself sipping on a cool tropical smoothie bursting with alkaline ingredients that give your body a boost.

Cleanses are most effective when you are dedicated and enjoying yourself. If you feel like you're suffering, you're more likely to break your diet or cleanse and go on a binge. The best thing to keep a cleanse from going south is variation. Try recipes that pique your interest and you are actually excited to try. Switch up your routine and challenge yourself to dry as many detoxifying recipes as you can within your 7 days cleanse. In the end, you can decide on the winner!

## Cleanse Kickstart

If you want to give you're cleanse an extra kickstart, keep a bottle of alkaline water with you to sip throughout the day. It will speed up the cleansing process and increase your daily hydration.  Ideally, you should take in about 1 liter of alkaline water every two hours to effectively flush out your system. Ginger tea is also a great detoxing beverage to take advantage of during your cleanse.

## A Cleanse Walkthrough

Here is an example of what your food intake should look like on a day of your cleanse:

- 8 am: Gulp down a big c of green juice or another raw ingredient smoothie. Emphasis is placed here on "raw." Raw vegetables and fruits contain the most alkaline benefits so to get that morning boost, stick to raw foods.

- 9 am sip a-c of ginger tea or alkaline water. Ginger is the best because it is highly alkalizing, but if ginger isn't your thing you can try a different kind of herbal tea. (Stay away from non-herbal blends!)
- 10 am: Enjoy a protein-filled "breakfast" smoothie. (Try the red velvet protein boost recipe!)
- 11am-12pm: By now you should be finished 1 liter of alkaline water.
- 12 pm: Make your lunch of choice, packed with raw alkaline foods of course! (Try the rainbow super salad or spicy summer soup recipe!)
- 1 pm: Sip a-c of ginger tea.
- 2 pm: Try another c of raw juice smoothie.
- 2pm-4pm: You should be finished drinking another 1 liter of alkaline water.
- 4 pm: Drink another c of a filling protein-heavy smoothie.
- 5 pm: Sip a-c of ginger tea.
- 6 pm: Make your dinner of choice. This can be the hardest meal to stick to your cleanse so try something fun and flavorful but still packed with raw

fruits and veggies like the roasted beet and lentil bowl paired with not your average tomato soup.

- 7pm-8pm: Finish off your last 1 liter of alkaline water.
- 9 pm: Sip a-c of ginger tea.
- 10pm-bedtime: If your tummy is still rumbling, munch on some veggie sticks or polish off some leftover juice/smoothie.

The first couple of days of your cleanse might result in headaches and low energy because of the drastic change in food intake. Be careful not to push yourself beyond your boundaries. Taking the first steps toward healthy living is an achievement in itself, so do not feel like you have to suffer for this to work. If you ever feel lightheaded or dizzy, do not be afraid to grab an extra snack or sneak in some extra protein (alkaline-based of course!) to keep your body happy. The most important part of this diet is to listen to your body. If your body is telling you "Woah Woah Woah we do not like that," listen to it and take a step back. Everybody's body is different and will adapt to this cleanse in a different way. Pay attention to the signs your body is sending you to cleanse in a safe and healthy way.

# Activity on a Cleanse

Another important thing to remember during this cleanse is that your body is used to taking in a significantly larger amount of calories, carbs, and fats. While this cleanses, in the long run, will drastically improve your energy levels, the first few days might leave you feeling weak and depleted. This is totally normal! Because of this, carefully monitor your activity level to keep from pushing yourself too far.

Light yoga and meditative breathing exercises are the perfect addition to keep you active during this cleanse. Not only will they give your body the activity it needs to stay healthy, but they are also a great way to really get into the mindset of healthy living and this cleanse. Center yourself on healthy bodily practices in mind and body for the full effect! The food we ingest leaves a mark on our body but so does our environment. High stress can contribute to faulty cell growth and high acid levels just as much as a bad diet does. Light exercise and stretching can combat this and change your whole mindset for a completely rounded health-conscious mind AND body.

Cleanses are exciting and may make you feel like you're on the track to a healthy pristine body. However, cleanses are an energy sap, especially because of low protein and carb intake. Our bodies feed off of those to provide energy, so without them, while your body is still transitioning, it can be tiring and discouraging. The right kind of activity though can enforce your cleanse and help move it along. Here are a couple of things to keep in mind when planning you're cleansing.

For running, rowing, cycling, and other endurance activities, you need a lot of solid food for your body to draw energy from. While it doesn't mean you have to leave these fitness habits behind when you start a cleanse, it means you have to be extra mindful of what your body is telling you. Fuel up with raw, solid veggies to keep yourself in the best shape possible.

For strength training, you will need protein-heavy foods so make sure to load up with a protein shake or nut bar before you head into a lifting session. Without protein, your body can't repair muscle strain and damage which poses a risk for injury.

For activities that increase your heart rate significantly like Pilates or swimming, so amp up the protein and superfood intake. Cardiovascular activities burn excess fat fast, but your body won't be able to stay energized without these additions. Otherwise, it will feel like running with chains on your ankles!

Remember, regardless of the activities you choose, listen to your body and keep it happy. That's the most important part of a cleanse! Happy body means happy you.

## Tips for success

*Don't let yourself get too hungry:* If you let yourself get to a point where you are not just a little hungry but are absolutely starving then it is going to be difficult for you to think rationally about what you are about to put into your body. Rather than looking for something healthy to eat you are going to be more concerned with eating something ASAP. As it doesn't take much of a slip to push you out of ketosis completely this can be a relatively dangerous position to let yourself fall into.

This is an easy scenario to prevent, however, as long as you take a little bit of extra time each day to plan ahead and ensure that you are always going to have something that is diet-friendly on hand. It is equally important that you try and guarantee that you don't skip meals and also eat at the same times every day. If your body gets into a routine then it will know what to expect, making it less likely that you will find yourself hungry unexpectedly with no way to satisfy your body's cravings.

*Stick to the three-color rule:* While following the alkaline diet can provide you with just as much variety as any other when you are just getting started it can be easy to find a few foods you enjoy and stick with them to the exclusion of all else. This means that if you are ever going to broaden your horizons you are going to want to make a point of eating something orange, something red and something green for every meal. Foods that contain these colors tend to be healthier than the alternatives and more filling as well. As an added bonus, foods in the three color groups are frequently credited with making those who consume them frequently look and feel younger as well.

*Have the right foods on hand at the right time:* When you are exercising regularly, it can be easy to get a little lax now and then when it comes to what you are eating exactly. However, if you use the fact that you exercise as an excuse to eat poorly, you will risk putting your health at risk, canceling out all of your hard work as a result. What's more, you will find that your overall results will be much improved if you make it a point of keeping enough healthy fats in your system to power your entire workout. Likewise, you are going to want to follow up with an exercise routine with extra protein to ensure your muscles have the tools they need to grow as a result.

Additionally, studies show that a longer, milder period of exercise burns the same number of calories as a short, intense workout, while also leaving you less hungry as a result. As such, if you stick to a more moderate workout you are less likely to feel the need to binge after the fact.

*Spice things up:* If you find yourself feeling hungry at the end of every meal, then your macros might not be to blame. Instead, you may be consuming less of the types of spices that generally help your body to know when it has had enough, leaving you feeling hungry despite the fact that you actually ate a full meal. Capsaicin spice, one of the most commonly used means of making food spicy, has the side effect of increasing the rate that endorphins are released from the body increasing the rate at which you feel full as a result. What's more, you can buy it as an additive and add a little bit of it to all of your meals, helping to train your body to your new way of eating more easily.

*Approach plateaus the right way:* Reach plateaus where your weight loss stalls out is a common part of any long-term weight loss plan. First and foremost, it is important to keep in mind that this is a natural part of the process which means there is no reason to let it get to you or cause you to do anything rash. Rapidly switching diets is only going to cause more harm every single time. Instead, try powering through the plateau by ensuring that you are sleeping at least eight hours per night.

*Don't rely on willpower early on*: While eventually, you will build up the willpower to make good decisions in the heat of the moment, the truth of the matter is that relying on your willpower early on is a recipe for disaster. Until you get the basics of the diet under your belt you are going to want to minimize how much you need to rely on willpower as much as possible if you hope to come out on top in the long run. Keep in mind that things like eating family-style, using large plates or even doing something besides eating while you are eating, are all going to make it more difficult for you to control yourself, and plan accordingly. This means that if there are multiple dietary options on the table, keep the serving dishes away from the table so you aren't tempted.

By removing willpower from the fact of whether or not you are going to lose weight, you will also eliminate much of the inherent shame and judgment you feel when you bring those issues to the fore. It is important to keep in mind that failing in this scenario is not a failure of you as a person, it is the failure of the system you have created for yourself. Putting new systems into place is a productive way to deal with these feelings, while at the same time making it easier for yourself to succeed in the future.

*Never skip a meal*: While it may seem to make sense that skipping the occasional meal should promote weight loss, after all, you are eating fewer calories in a given day, the fact is the opposite is true. This is because your body gets into a habit of taking in and burning calories throughout the day based on your average eating patterns and missing a meal gums up the works. Rather than taking in and burning calories as anticipated, your body now needs to stretch what was already available further than it was planning to which means it will have to play catchup later on. This, in turn, means that skipping that meal will likely cause you to hold onto more weight that day, not less as your body will try and hold onto everything it can until it knows just what is going on.

You should always start your day off with a healthy and nutritious breakfast as this will kick your metabolism into gear at the start of the day, keeping it in the habit of not holding onto any additional fat throughout the day. Ideally, you will want to split your day up into three moderate meals and then three light snacks so that you are eating about every three hours. This will ensure that once your metabolism gets going in the morning, it won't stop, burning more calories overall throughout the day than you would otherwise. It is important to watch what you consume with this strategy, however, as choosing unhealthy snacks will negate any work that you are doing by sticking to the diet.

*Set the right goals:* Once you do start your new diet, you are going to want to take into account that a 3,500-calorie deficit is going to lead to the loss of one pound of fat, but that this equation doesn't take muscle growth into the equation at all. This means that if you are exercising regularly then you may end up losing less weight per week, but still end up looking and feeling better regardless. If you find yourself feeling discouraged based on the results from the scale it is important to consider how long it took you to reach your current weight and fitness level and then give yourself a comparable period of time to get back to where you need to be. Getting to your current point didn't happen overnight and there is no reason to expect to change things up drastically will lead to overnight results either.

*Drink more water:* Since you are adding new habits to your repertoire anyway, it is a good idea to add drinking more water to the list. Specifically, you should aim for about 64 ounces of water per day, to ensure your body has all the water it needs to operate at maximum efficiency. If you live in a warm, dry climate, or exercise regularly you are going to want to aim even higher and try and consume a gallon of water per day. If you don't drink that much water naturally or don't believe you need to drink the recommended amount, give it a try for a few weeks and you will be surprised by the results.

Specifically, you will be surprised at how frequently your body was sending you signals saying it was hungry when in reality it was just looking for something to drink. Drinking the right amount of water per day will also provide your metabolism with the boost that it needs to function in peak form and ensure you lose as much weight each week as possible.

*Don't let yourself make excuses:* While it is important to not get started on a new diet when your schedule is extremely busy or you have extra stress or anxiety on your plate, it is also important to not keep putting it off every time something new comes up. Life is always going to be busy, and at some point, the reasons you have for crying off are simply going to be excused to avoid getting started. Be frank with yourself and understand that there are always going to be something standing in your way from making positive life changes, you simply need to power through them if you ever hope to see real success.

At some point, all you can do is say enough is enough and get down to business. After all, the only person that can really motivate you to stick with a healthy diet in the long term is you. This is why it is so important to not let yourself down. If you truly commit to finding personal success when it comes to your weight loss goals then there should be nothing that can stop you. It really is as simple as that.

# Herbal Medicine

More and more people turn to herbal medicine each year, and it is no surprise. Humans have been mastering the benefits of nature for years now, since the beginning of civilization. Hieroglyphs from Ancient Egypt depict the use of natural healing remedies, and there is mention of these remedies also in Chinese scripture. Many countries still use traditional medicine as a go-to, and it is not just underdeveloped countries. Herbal remedies are used in Africa and Native American tribes during healing rituals, and large, wealthy countries like China have integrated herbal medicine into their traditional medical system.

Herbal medicine has hit the United States by storm too. In the last couple of decades, the general public has been struggling with the inflated prices of over-the-counter medicines, and natural remedies are making a comeback. More people are turning away from processed products and attempting to take a step towards natural living. Organic product sales have exploded in the states, herbal medicine included.

People who wish to take a step towards living naturally have been choosing to cut out the pharmaceutical chemicals in exchange for herbal medicine. Natural medicine is a healthy choice, not simply a placebo. Natural resources have kept humans alive and healthy for centuries, curing ailments of all kinds from chronic pain to diseases. In ancient times, pharmaceutical drugs didn't exist so humans did what they could to learn about the land around them. In doing so they discovered one of the earth's treasures: healing. Ever since then we have been utilizing what we can from around us.

## Why Use Herbal Medicine?

When switching to an alkaline diet, it is a good idea to also adopt herbal medicine practice to keep up your all-natural, non-processed habit. Herbal medicine is any product made from plants and botanicals to aid in maintaining bodily health. For a plant to be considered medicinal, it must yield healing or therapeutic effects. They work by naturally synthesizing secondary metabolites in the body, working with the body's natural system to heal and take away the pain.

Herbal medicine is most effective in treating chronic pain and preventing illnesses. For immediate health concerns or emergencies, herbal treatment falls short. However, using this natural form of treatment is a great way to cut excess chemicals out of your daily routine. Many people turn to herbs for a natural way to heal bodily harm without their wallet taking a hit.

Though many over the counter medications are also plant-based, it is often mixed with other chemical solutions rather than pure plant substances like herbal medicine. Studies have shown that it is more beneficial to use herbal medicines to consume the active healing ingredient in herbs rather than using over the counter pharmaceuticals that isolate the active ingredient. This is because when isolated, the active ingredients used can cause more severe side effects. For example, meadowsweet contains salicylic acid, an ingredient used in aspirin. A side effect of aspirin is stomach bleeding, a condition that is not caused by meadowsweet as a whole. Meadowsweet contains natural combs. that prevent the irritation that results in stomach bleeding. The downside of consuming active healing ingredients like this though is that it can be hard to tell the exact dosage of active ingredients in each set of herbs. However, this factor is safer by a large margin than the risk of harmful side effects.

People have been turning to herbal medicine not only because of its natural healing properties but also because of economic factors. Pharmaceuticals, even with insurance, are extremely pricey and can make a huge dent in your wallet, especially with chronic illnesses. If you suffer from chronic pain or wish to maintain a healthy body by taking preventative measures, that is a lot of trips to the pharmacy and a lot of money spent. Luckily for you, herbal medicine is the perfect fix for this. You can buy exactly what you need in the amount you need from a wider variety of stores. It is also cheaper and will not affect your insurance rate.

You can see why this form of traditional medicine is still widely used across the globe. Many countries don't have proper healthcare, so herbal medicine is sometimes the only option for those who can't afford a trip to the pharmacy. It is also cost-effective in that it doesn't take a trip to the doctors to obtain. Of course, you should consult a professional before using any medication, but herbal therapists are easy to find and charge way less than a general practitioner will.

Don't be fooled, though. Herbal medicine is not just used by the poor and not so well-off. It makes sense to partake in a cost-effective treatment program that is personalized to each individual. China, one of the most successful economies in the world currently, has an established system of traditional natural medicine. They do not use them because they do not have access to pharmaceutical drugs, but rather that herbal medicine presents a way to heal long-term problems naturally in a cost-effective way.

Think of it this way. If you walked into a store and saw two of the same items on a shelf priced differently, would you get the more expensive one? No, that would just be silly. Now imagine the more expensive version of the same item is also soaked in chemicals with detrimental side effects. Add on the fact that you have to go to the store every week to get this item. Unless the item is one of a kind and will change your life (like serious illness treatment), wouldn't you choose the natural, easier, cost-effective route?

## Forms of Herbal Medicine

Herbal medicine comes in many different forms, depending on what ailment you wish to treat. There are powders, pills, capsules, and liquids galore, and these medicines can be taken a variety of different ways. An added bonus of herbal medicine is the ease in which it can be used. Pills, of course, are an option, but you can also brew herbal blends in your tea, add them to a bath, or use an herbal moisturizer or lotion.

This form of treatment is natural and easy to use, but it does not come without its difficulties. Herbal medicine can react badly with over the counter prescriptions so it is important to educate yourself and consult a doctor before self-administering treatment. Just because it is natural does not mean that it is not potent, so herbal medicines aren't anything to play around with.

Consult a medical professional before using these suggested doses:

- Teas: 1 c, 4x a day
- Powdered: 2-4 capsules, 3x a day
- Tinctures: 2-4 drops, 3x a day
- Extracts: 1 tablet, 3x a day

For chronic or acute pain, pills and liquids or oils are the best to use because they are prepared in a way that ensures the potency of the herb's active ingredient is strong. These forms of treatment will result in the most immediate relief for bothersome symptoms.

For preventative steps, turn to herbal teas, baths, and lotions. These forms are easy to incorporate into your daily routine and are great to have on hand in the house. They are not as potent and can work more slowly, but the ease of use for these make them the perfect preventative measure for illness and pain.

## What To Use

Unsure of what treats what? Consult this chart of common ailments to find the perfect herbal treatment for you. Medicinal herb labels will not list a specific ailment or treatment because of the way they are regulated. Herbs do not go through clinical trials or medicinal manufacturing standards so the label cannot claim to be a specific treatment. For example, a label on St. John's wort, an herb known to be used to treat depression, will read "uplifts mood" rather than an antidepressant. Again, it is important to understand that this list is not a substitute for a medical professional, and you should take care to look into the side effects and consult a professional before using.

| Ailment | Herbal Medicine |
| --- | --- |
| Allergies | Cayenne, nettle herb, garlic |
| Anxiety | Poppy |
| Arthritis | Yucca, ginger, devil's claw |
| Bladder Infection | Cranberry, Pipsissewa, marshmallow root |
| Rashes | St. John's wort cream, chamomile |
| Sinus | Eucalyptus, eyebright, cayenne |
| Cough | Wild cherry bark, licorice root, sage |
| Cold | Elderberries, ginger, sage |
| Depression | St. John's wort |
| Headaches | Meadowsweet, feverfew, willow bark |
| Insomnia | Chamomile, valerian, poppy |
| Premenstrual syndrome | Evening primrose |
| Stomachache | Peppermint, ginger |
| Memory loss | Ginkgo Biloba |

| Stress | Ginseng |
|---|---|
| High blood pressure | Hawthorn |
| Painful menstruation/vaginitis | Black cohosh |

## Get the Most Out of Your Products

Within the past few years, the World Health Organization has concluded that over 80% of the world depends on herbal medicine for some portion of their health care. With the popularity of herbal medicine increasing, the market is growing and may seem unnavigable to new herbal users. Herbal medicine is not considered a drug by the FDA; it is considered a food, so it pays to learn how to get the most out of your product.

The most important thing is to do your research before. It is easy to get overwhelmed staring at a wall full of hundreds of different labels and brands. Decide what you need before you go to the store to save yourself the headache. You should, of course, consult with your medical practitioner before using herbal medicine, but if you are unable to access a medical professional, take your time and find a credible source to refer to.

We've mentioned the various forms that herbal medicine can take which has the potential to become another never-ending question for people new to natural remedies. Not surprisingly, there isn't a cure-all solution. The form of medicine you should pick depends entirely on you and the ailment you wish to treat because each variety is going to have a different level of potency.

For long-term treatment of ailments such as chronic pain, extracts are your best friend. In this form, the herbs ingredients are kept stable and active almost indefinitely. Extracts can come in liquid or solid tablet form. Tinctures are similar to extracts, just slightly less potent. They come in liquid form, but they often contain less active plant ingredients and more alcohol. Though tinctures can be potent and helpful, they are alcohol-based, so it is best to steer clear of these while on your alkaline diet.

Powdered herbs and teas are convenient, but are much less potent than extracts and tinctures and run the risk of being completely inactive. For these forms, herbs are often bulk dried and ground which rapidly increases the rate of oxidation. Sniff check before you buy! As strange as it may sound at first, sniffing your herbs can be a great way to determine if they are still active because inactive herbs lose their color and odor.

Steer clear of everything but the kitchen sink mixes that claim to treat all ailments. Mixing these herbs could have bad side effects as not every plant has been studied with how they react with other plants. For example, St. John's wort should never be taken with other medicines. As always, check with a medical professional before using any of these medicines, but as a general rule, stay away from mixes.

You'll also want to stay away from overseas products without extensive research. Not that imported products can't be equally as quality, but different countries have different standards for manufacturing. This means that you could end up with a product containing significantly different doses of active ingredients, or the herb could be cut with an unknown chemical. Also, because the fresher the herb the better its healing properties, overseas products can get dicey due to the time it takes to transport, the use of preservatives, and bulk packaging.

Though herbal medicine isn't as heavily regulated like pharmaceuticals, there are still ways to make sure that you are getting what you are paying for. Stick to brands labeled "standardized". This label means that the medication has been tested to ensure a certain level of the plant's active ingredient is present. Research reputable brands and check for the sticker for the best product. Regardless of brands, research, or correct labels, the most important thing is to use common sense. do not take these herbal medicines lightly. Some are just as potent as pharmaceutical medicines. Listen to your body, and stick to a low dosage to start with. If any side effects pop up, stop using the herb and speak to a professional.

## Essential Oils: Hitting the World by Storm

Essential oils are a form of herbal medicine that has hit the world by storm. Almost every store has a version of a diffuser on sale, and various essential oil blends decorate the shelves of hundreds of home and beauty stores. The natural remedy trend has taken over the country, and there is a good reason why. The benefits of herbal medicine are clear, but most importantly, essential oils are easy to diffuse and forget about, filling your home with beautiful fresh scents.

Beware of phony mixes though. As the popularity of essential oils grows, so does the consumerism market, meaning that some brands are going to be better quality than others. It is important that the herb's healing ingredients are active for its health benefits. The easiest way to ensure this is by purchasing pure oils, not mixed blends. Make the healing combinations on your own with the pure oil to ensure that the healing ingredients are active.

Try out some of these combinations!

For focus:
- 2 drops of peppermint
- 2 drops of lemon
- 1 drop of basil

- 2 drops of grapefruit
- 2 drops of lavender
- 1 drop of rosemary

For stress relief:

- 2 drops of roman chamomile
- 3 drops of lavender
- 2 drops of ylang-ylang

For calm:

- 3 drops of lime
- 3 drops of mandarin
- 3 drops of lavender

For energy:

- 3 drops of peppermint
- 3 drops of lemon
- 3 drops of rosemary

For a wakeup boost:

- 4 drops of peppermint
- 4 drops wild of orange

For happiness:

- 2 drops of wild orange
- 2 drops of lime
- 2 drops of peppermint
- 2 drops of frankincense

For an immune system boost:

- 2 drops of clove
- 2 drops of wild orange
- 2 drops of rosemary
- 2 drops of cinnamon
- 2 drops of eucalyptus

For sleep:

- 3 drops of juniper berry
- 3 drops of lavender
- 3 drops of roman chamomile

For headache relief:

- 2 drops of peppermint
- 2 drops of thyme
- 2 drops of lavender
- 2 drops of rosemary
- 2 drops of marjoram

For a cold:

- 2 drops of lemon
- 4 drops of peppermint
- 5 drops of rosemary
- 4 drops of eucalyptus
- 3 drops of cypress

For a brain boost:

- 4 drops of cinnamon
- 2 drops of rosemary
- 4 drops of peppermint

Purchase a diffuser almost anywhere and follow the manufacturer's directions for adding water and turning it on. Then use any one of these oil blends to see what all the hype is about!

# Breakfast and Brunch

Keeping to your alkaline diet with a busy schedule can be hard, especially when you're in a rush to get out of the house and do not know what to grab. This can be dangerous to your diet because breakfast foods tend to be sugary and processed or full of greasy acidic foods that will throw off your healthy habits. Not to fear! This chapter includes a number of breakfast and brunch recipes that are easy to make ahead and then grab and go. They are all alkalizing yet delicious so you do not have to sacrifice taste for health!

# Berry Breakfast Bowl

A quick and easy breakfast for people with a sweet tooth, this recipe is light yet flavorful! You can substitute any of these fruits for your personal favorites. Experiment and see which combination you like best!

Total Prep and Cooking Time: 15 min.
Difficulty Level: Easy
Yields: 4 Servings

## Ingredients:

Banana - 1 c

Papaya - 2 c

Strawberries - 2 c

Dried cranberries - 2 T

Raspberries - 1 c

Blueberries - 1 c

Dried, unsweetened coconut flakes - 1 T

Walnuts - 2 T

Agave - 2 T

## Instructions:

Mix the berries and sliced fruit in a medium bowl gently so you do not mush the fruit.

Pour agave over the fruit, and stir the mix again gently.

Sprinkle coconut, walnuts, and cranberries over the mixed fruit bowl.

Serve and enjoy!

# Hearty Sweet Potato Toast

Calling all sweet potatoes lovers! This recipe is quick and easy to adjust with your personal favorite flavors. Top your slices with this sweet concoction, or try your hand at coming up with your own.

Total Prep and Cooking Time: 15 min.

Difficulty Level: Easy

Yields: 4 Servings

**Ingredients:**

Almond butter - 2 T

Granola - 0.5 c

Hemp seeds - 1 T

Sweet potato - 1 whole

Coconut oil - 2 T

Salt and pepper - To Taste

Also needed: baking sheet

**Instructions:**

Preheat your oven to 425 degrees while you grease a large baking sheet.

Wash the sweet potato and cut it into slices that are about ¼ of an inch thick.

Evenly coat both sides of the potato slices in coconut oil, sprinkling with salt and pepper to taste.

Place the slices on a greased baking sheet about an inch apart.

Toss your potatoes in the oven for 15-20 minutes. They are done when you are able to  lightly pierce them with a fork.

Cool potato pieces on a rack before topping them.

Once cooled, spread the almond butter over the crispy pieces of sweet potato.

Sprinkle on the granola and hemp seeds.

Serve and enjoy!

## Butternut Waffles

If you're missing a full breakfast ensemble by switching your diet to alkaline, try this recipe to cure some of your cravings. It is great for a special brunch treat!

Total Prep and Cooking Time: 45 min.
Difficulty Level: Intermediate
Yields: 8 Waffles

## Ingredients:

Pumpkin pie spice - 1 tsp.

Almond milk - 1.5 c

Baking powder - 1 T

White whole wheat flour - 2 c

Salt - 0.5 tsp.

Butternut squash puree - 1.25 c

Maple syrup - 0.25 c

Coconut oil - 0.5 c

Egg whites - 2 large

Banana - 0.5 c mashed

Chopped pecans - 1 c

Also needed: waffle iron

**Instructions:**

Whisk together the flour, pumpkin pie spice, baking powder, and salt in a large bowl.

In a separate bowl, mix the almond milk, squash, banana, coconut oil, and maple syrup.

Combine the wet and dry ingredients.

Whip the separated egg whites with a whisk or hand mixer in a separate bowl until stiff peaks form.

Fold the egg whites into the batter until it is partially mixed in and fluffy.

Preheat the waffle iron.

Pour about 0.5 c of batter onto the waffle iron and cook until golden brown.

Serve with maple syrup and chopped pecans.

# Mini Veggie Quiche

Easy to make and even easier to take on the go, these mini quiche care a must-have for busy bees that have to rush out the door in the morning.

Total Prep and Cooking Time: 45 min.
Difficulty Level: Easy
Yields: 6 Servings

**Ingredients:**

Eggs whites- 3

Chopped peppers - 0.5 c

Wonton wrappers - 12

Spinach - 0.5 c

Almond milk - 0.25 c

Salt and pepper - To Taste

Also needed: muffin tin

**Instructions:**

Spray your muffin tin with non-stick spray while preheating your oven to 350 degrees.

Overlap two wonton wrappers in each c so that most of the pan is covered.

Whisk the egg whites, almond milk, spinach, and peppers together in a medium bowl, adding salt or pepper to taste.

Pour the egg mixture equally into the muffin tin. Each c should be about 0.75 of the way full.

Bake in preheated oven for 20-25 minutes. The center should be completely set.

Let quiche c cool for 5-10 minutes in the pan before removing to serve.

## Very Berry Muffins

Unwrap some yummy goodness with this recipe for mixed berry muffins. They are easy to bake and the perfect sized for a sweet bite in the morning.

Total Prep and Cooking Time: 45 min.

Difficulty Level: Easy

Yields: 6 Servings

### Ingredients:

Chickpea flour - 1 c

Spelt flour - 0.75 c + 1 T

Grapeseed oil - 2 T

Water - 0.75 c

Agave - 6 T

Blueberries - 1 c

Salt - 0.5 tsp.

Also needed: muffin tin

**Instructions:**

Preheat your oven to 350 degrees and spray muffin tin with non-stick spray.

Mix the flour, oil, water, agave, blueberries, and salt together until the batter is smooth.

Pour the batter equally into the six c of the muffin tin.

Bake in preheated oven for 30 minutes. Let the tin cool for 10 minutes before removing and serving.

# Pumpkin Pie French Toast

For a warm breakfast perfect for chilly autumn Saturdays, try this recipe for pumpkin pie French toast. It will have you itching to jump in a pile of leaves or carve a pumpkin!

Total Prep and Cooking Time: 30 min.

Difficulty Level: Easy

Yields: 4 Servings

## Ingredients:

Almond milk - 0.75 c

Gluten-free bread - 8 slices

Pumpkin puree - 0.5 c

Nutmeg - 0.25 tsp.

Cinnamon - 1 tsp.

Maple syrup - 1 T

Almond milk - 0.25 c

Sea salt - 0.25 tsp.

Coconut oil - 1 tsp.

Also needed: baking sheet

**Instructions:**

Whisk the almond milk, maple syrup, pumpkin puree, nutmeg, salt, and cinnamon together in a bowl.

Spread gluten-free bread out onto the baking tray.

Pour pumpkin mixture over the slices of bread, making sure to spread and coat all the sides.

Put a non-stick pan on medium heat and grease with the coconut oil.

Place the slices of bread in the pan and cook for 3 minutes on each side or until golden brown. Be careful to reduce heat as needed to prevent burning.

Drizzle with maple syrup and serve!

# Loaded Veggie Breakfast Casserole

Having people over for brunch but do not want to ruin your alkaline diet? Use this veggie casserole recipe to wow your guests without sacrificing your diet.

Total Prep and Cooking Time: 55 min.

Difficulty Level: Intermediate

Yields: 8 Servings

## Ingredients:

Baby spinach - 3 c

Green onion - 0.25 c chopped

Basil leaves - 3 T

Yellow onions - 2 chopped

Tomatoes - 2 chopped

Broccoli florets - 2.5 c

Avocados - 2 cubed

Egg whites - 12

Sea salt - 1 tsp.

Coconut oil - 4 T

Eggplant - 1 large

Also needed: 9x14 casserole dish

**Instructions:**

Grease your casserole dish while preheating the oven to
450 degrees.

Slice large eggplant into a quarter of an inch thick slices,
and lay them in the casserole dish so there is a completely
covered layer. Drizzle half of the coconut oil over all the
slices.

Put the eggplant slices in the oven and cook until golden
brown - about 20 minutes.

 Put a skillet on medium heat with the rest of the coconut
oil. Simmer the onions and broccoli florets in the pan for 5
minutes.

Add the basil, spinach, and green onion to the pan and cook
until the spinach wilts.

Remove the pan from the heat and stir in the tomatoes,
avocado, and salt.

Combine the egg whites in a medium bowl.

Take the casserole out of the oven and pour the veggie
mixture over the eggplant. Add the egg white mixture last.

Reduce the oven temperature to 400 degrees. Put the
casserole dish back in the oven and cook for 35 minutes.

Insert a toothpick in the center and check if it comes out
clean to know it is done.

 Cut into squares and serve!

# Quick and Easy "Oatmeal"

This mock oatmeal recipe is great for those on the go who want a quick breakfast solution without the loss of nutrition. This hearty dish will stick to your bones and give you that boost of energy to tackle a big day!

Total Prep and Cooking Time: 10 min.

Difficulty Level: Easy

Yields: 2 Servings

## Ingredients:

Chia seeds - 2 T

Almond milk - 0.5 c

Quinoa flakes - 1 c

Cinnamon - 0.5 T

Coconut oil - 2 T

Stevia - 1 T

Walnuts - 1 c crushed

## Instructions:

The night before soak chia seeds in about 2 T of water.

Microwave quinoa flakes for 3 minutes with 1 c of water.

Pour the chia seeds into the quinoa flakes.

Add stevia, almond milk, cinnamon, and coconut oil and stir until evenly mixed.

Sprinkle walnuts on top or drizzle with honey and enjoy.

# Sweet Southern Egg C

These egg c may seem plain at first glance but they pack a punch! This breakfast is easy and great for on-the-go eats.

Total Prep and Cooking Time: 45 min.

Difficulty Level: Intermediate

Yields: 12 Servings

## Ingredients:

Eggs whites- 12 large

Sweet potato - 1 c grated

Coconut oil - 2 T

Kale - 2 c

Salt - 0.5 tsp.

Also needed: 12-muffin tin

## Instructions:

Start by preheating your oven to 375 degrees.

Put a large pan over medium heat with the coconut oil. Stir in the kale and simmer for about 5 minutes until it is wilted.

Toss in the grated sweet potatoes and sprinkle with half of the salt. Cook for 10 minutes, stirring occasionally.

Set mixture aside to cool.

Whisk together your egg whites with the rest of the salt.

Fold your veggie mixture into the egg whites.

Grease your muffin tin and fill each c completely with the egg mixture.

Bake until the center of the egg is puffed up - about 20-25 minutes - and set aside to cool.

Serve right away or seal in a refrigerated container for up to 3 days.

# Chickpea Frittata

Eggs are breakfast staple, but in large quantities, they pose a risk to your alkaline eating habits. Try out this recipe for a frittata that won't ruin your diet but will fill the egg-sized hole in your heart.

Total Prep and Cooking Time: 30 min.
Difficulty Level: Easy
Yields: 4 Servings

## Ingredients:

Broccoli - 2 c sliced

Scallions - 0.5 c

Alkaline water - 1.75 c

Garbanzo bean flour - 0.5 c

Coconut oil - 1 T

## Instructions:

Put a pan on medium heat with the coconut oil. Sauté your veggies until they are slightly browned.

In a large bowl, combine the garbanzo bean flour and the alkaline water. Mix until the batter is smooth.

Pour the batter over the cooked vegetables and cook until the center is firm.

Add salt and pepper to your preference.

Slice your frittata into wedges and serve.

## On-The-Go Breakfast Pudding

Sweet fruits, protein, and ready to grab and go. What more could you want? This chia pudding is the perfect amount of a deliciously creamy breakfast that will keep you healthy and energized all day!

Total Prep and Cooking Time: 10 min.

Difficulty Level: Easy

Yields: 1 Serving

### Ingredients:

Soaked almonds - 2 T

Chia seeds - 0.25 c

Vanilla extract - 0.5 tsp.

Almond milk - 1 c

Blueberries - 0.5 c

Stevia - 1 tsp.

### Instructions:

Combine all your ingredients into a medium bowl and mix until everything seems evenly distributed.

Pour your mixture into a mason jar or to-go bowl and place in the fridge to chill overnight. The chia seeds will expand and soften as they chill, soaking up the liquid to make a pudding-like consistency.

Pull out the next morning to enjoy a stress-free start.

# Appetizers

Make your meal special and unique by adding one of these appetizer recipes. Full of alkalizing nutrients, these recipes pack a punch! They are fresh and flavorful so you and your guests probably won't even notice you're being healthy. Skip the processed cheese dips and chips and try these out instead!

# Spring Rolls

These spring rolls are fresh and light, the perfect appetizer to put that special touch on a meal. Try out this rainbow recipe!

Total Prep and Cooking Time: 20 min.
Difficulty Level: Easy
Yields: 5 Servings

## Ingredients:

Rice papers - 5

Basil - 0.25 c

Spinach - 1 c

Arugula - 0.5 c

Carrot - 1 c shredded

Avocado - 1 c sliced

Olives - 0.5 c

## Instructions:

Chop all your veggies up finely and put them aside.

Fill a flat dish with warm water about one inch deep.

Place your rice papers in the dish one at a time for about five seconds until the entire sheet is coated in water and softened.

Spread out your softened rice paper sheet on a plate.

Stack your desired combination of veggie slices in the center of the rice paper. Use about half as much as you think you would need. It is important not to overfill or the rice papers might tear.

Fold two opposite edges toward the center and roll the rest of it up to form a spring roll.

Repeat the previous steps for the rest of the rice papers and chopped veggies.

Serve and enjoy!

## "Taco" Dip

A party seems incomplete without taco dip. Try this alkaline-style "taco" dip for a delicious way to stay on a healthy track without having to miss out.

Total Prep and Cooking Time: 20 min.

Difficulty Level: Intermediate

Yields: 6 Servings

## Ingredients:

Sprouted grain tortillas - 6 tortillas

Water - 0.25 c

Taco seasoning - 1 package

Garlic - 2 cloves minced

Carrots - 1 c diced

White onion - 0.5 c diced

Tempeh - 1 block

Cherry tomatoes - 1 c halved

Coconut oil - 2 T

Scallions - 2 T chopped

Chives - 2 T chopped

Cilantro - 2 T chopped

Sea salt - 0.5 tsp.

**Instructions:**

Use a food grater to shred your tempeh block so that it resembles a ground beef consistency.

Put a pan on medium heat and douse with the coconut oil. Throw in the onions and carrots and cook them until they are just a little bit soft.

Add in the garlic and cherry tomatoes and cook them for another 3 minutes while occasionally stirring. Make sure to cover your pan to use the heat to steam and cook your veggies.

Sprinkle your taco seasoning onto the veggie mix and then stir as you gradually add the water until everything is evenly mixed.

Toss in your grated tempeh and cover the pan to let the mixture cook for two more minutes.

Add in your herbs and stir well so that everything is well seasoned and evenly distributed. Remove your pan from the stove and set it aside.

Slice your tortillas into wedges that resemble chips and lightly toast them until they become crunchy. You can sprinkle your desired salt and herbs over them to give them an extra kick.

Serve your "taco" dip with the chips for scooping and enjoy!

## Tabbouleh Spread

This fresh tabbouleh salad is a delicious herby add-on to any dip spread. it is a good thing this dip is fresh and healthy because you won't be able to get enough of it!

Total Prep and Cooking Time: 20 min.

Difficulty Level: Easy

Yields: 6 Servings

## Ingredients:

Tomatoes - 2 medium chopped

Mint - 0.5 c chopped

Curly parsley - 1 c chopped

Prepared pearl quinoa - 2 c

Olive oil - 3 T

Lemon juice - 3 T

Salt and pepper - To Taste

## Instructions:

Wash your quinoa under cold water and cook it using the manufacturer's directions. Once cooked place the quinoa aside in a large bowl to cool.

Mix together your finely chopped mint and parsley before adding it to the cooked quinoa.

Toss in your chunky tomatoes and sprinkle the bowl with your desired amount of salt and pepper.

Whisk your oil and lemon juice in a separate small bowl until they are thoroughly combined. Pour the liquid over your quinoa mixture.

Stir your tabbouleh mixture well and serve with veggie slices or sprouted grain tortilla chips.

## Cucumber Hummus Sliders

These cucumber sliders are a perfect bite-sized appetizer to start off any gathering. They are especially good as a refreshing light bite in the summer and are just so darned cute!

Total Prep and Cooking Time: 15 min.
Difficulty Level: Easy
Yields: 10 Servings

### Ingredients:

Hummus - 1 c
Cucumber - 4 large
Parsley - 1 T

### Instructions:

Slice the rounded ends off of your cucumbers and cut them into ¼ of an inch slice.

Scoop out the seeds in the center of the cucumber slices but be careful not to break the thin bottom layer or else the hummus will fall through.

Let the cucumbers drain on a paper towel for about 5 minutes until the extra moisture is gone.

Spoon a small amount of hummus onto each cucumber and sprinkle parsley to top.

Serve and enjoy!

# Stuffed Mushrooms

Try out this recipe to serve your guests for an upscale appetizer without the stress. A bite out of the stuffed mushroom caps will surely impress!

Total Prep and Cooking Time: 15 min.

Difficulty Level: Easy

Yields: 10 Servings

**Ingredients:**

Cooked quinoa - 1 c

Red bell pepper - 0.25 c chopped

Brazil nut cheese - 0.5 c

Mushrooms - 10 whole

Sea salt - 0.25 tsp.

Vegetable broth - 2 c

Scallions - 0.25 c

Also needed: baking sheet

**Instructions:**

While you grease a baking sheet, preheat your oven to 350 degrees.

Wash your quinoa and cook to manufacturer's instructions in the vegetable broth until the liquid is completely absorbed.

Remove the mushroom stems, being careful not to break the "cap" part of the mushroom, and let them sit in warmed vegetable broth for 5 minutes.

Spread out the mushrooms on the baking sheet, leaving room between each of them.

Once the quinoa is finished cooking, mix in the bell peppers and nut cheese. Make sure the mix is evenly distributed.

Use a spoon to scoop out a small amount of quinoa and stuff your mushroom caps until they are nearly spilling over.

Place the baking tray in the oven for 10 minutes.

Remove your mushrooms when the edges are slightly browned and sprinkle them with scallions before serving.

# Four Layer Mediterranean Dip

This dish may look complicated at first glance but it is as easy as pressing start on the food processor. Try this recipe for an easy crowd-pleaser that is bright, unique, and flavorful. Step aside layered Mexican dip!

Total Prep and Cooking Time: 15 min.

Difficulty Level: Easy

Yields: 6 c/25 servings

## Ingredients:

Bottom Layer

Garlic - 1 clove

Olive oil - 0.5 c

Kalamata olives - 0.5 c pitted

Lentils - 0.5 c

Water - 1 c

Parsley - 0.25 c chopped

Salt - 0.25 tsp.

Second layer

Shallot - 2 T chopped

Zucchini - 0.5 c diced

Cashews - 0.5 c soaked

Garlic - 1 clove chopped

Basil - 0.5 c

Parsley - 0.25 c

Lemon juice - 1 T

Olive oil - 0.25 c

Water - 2 T

Third Layer

Cannellini beans - 28 oz.

Olive oil - 0.5 c

Rosemary - 1 large sprig

Garlic - 1 clove

Final Layer

Roasted red peppers - 1 c

Pine nuts - 0.25 c

Basil - 10 leaves minced

Cherry tomatoes - 1 pint quartered


Also needed: Deep dip dish

**Instructions:**

Begin on the first layer by bringing a pot with the water and lentils to a boil. Continue to simmer for 20 minutes until almost all of the water is absorbed.

Pour the lentils into a food processor and add the rest of the first layer ingredients. Pulse until the mixture is textured but evenly combined.

Spread the olive and lentil layer in the bottom of the dip dish.

Begin on the next layer of your dip by tossing all of the second layer's ingredients into the food processor. (Wash the appliance between dip layers.) Pulse until the mixture is creamy and very smooth.

Spoon the creamy basil layer onto the lentil layer and spread until it is even.

Start the third layer of dip by again putting all of the ingredients listed into the food processor. Pulse until the mixture is smooth and resembles the consistency of refried beans.

Sprinkle the roasted peppers over the creamy basil layer until the surface is evenly covered.

Spread the white bean layer on top of the roasted red peppers, making sure the surface is flat and even. Be gentle when spreading the bean dip so as not to shake around the red peppers.

Sprinkle the cherry tomatoes, basil, and pine nuts on top of the white bean layer to top it.

Serve with your favorite veggie sticks!

# Roasted Veggie Kabobs

These kabobs look brick roasted and taste just as good without all the hassle. This recipe is for fun light bites that are delicious and nutritious!

Total Prep and Cooking Time: 30 min.
Difficulty Level: Easy
Yields: 6 Servings

**Ingredients:**
Cherry tomatoes - 12
Zucchini - 2 large
White onion - 1 large
Olive oil - 0.25 c
Garlic - 3 cloves
Sea salt - To Taste
Garlic basil dip - 2 c
Pistachio nuts - 0.5 c
Basil - 1 c
Olive oil - 0.5 c
Garlic - 2 cloves
Zucchini - 1 c diced

Also needed: 6" skewers - 12

**Instructions:**

Preheat your oven to 400 degrees while lining a baking sheet with parchment.

Mix up the garlic and olive oil to set aside.

Chop up your veggies to begin to make the skewers. The zucchini should be cut into 0.5-inch rounds and the onions should be cut into large square chunks. Keep your cherry tomatoes whole.

Start making your kabobs by sliding the veggies onto the 6" skewers. Choose your own desired pattern (ex: zucchini, onion, tomato, onion, tomato, and zucchini).

Slather your kabobs with a generous amount of the mixed garlic oil and sprinkle them with your desired amount of salt.

Place the baking sheet into the oven and roast your veggies for 16 minutes until they are slightly crispy at the edges.

Use the baking time to make your garlicky basil dip by tossing all your dip ingredients into a blender or food processor and pulsing until the mixture is smooth. You can add more olive oil if the mixture is too dry and chunky.

Pull the veggies out of the oven and serve on a platter whole. Half the fun of this tasty appetizer is eating them off the stick! Serve with the garlicky basil dip and enjoy!

# Marrakesh Moroccan Eggplant Dip

Try a taste of Morocco with this rich cumin flavored eggplant dip. Scoop up as much as you can with crispy homemade chips before it is all gone!

Total Prep and Cooking Time: 40 min.

Difficulty Level: Easy

Yields: 6 Servings

## Ingredients:

Garlic - 4 cloves crushed

Lemon juice - 1 T

Olive oil - 2.5 T

Eggplant - 6 medium

Cumin - 1.5 tsp.

Sea salt - 3.25 tsp.

Sprouted grain tortilla wraps - 6 wraps

Also needed: 3 baking sheets

**Instructions:**

Preheat your oven to 375 degrees while lining 2 baking sheets with parchment paper.

Take your eggplants and trim the ends before cutting them in half lengthwise. Lay them face down on the baking sheets.

Poke tiny holes in the eggplant halves using a toothpick to allow the steam to escape while the eggplant cooks.

Place the 2 baking sheets with the eggplant in the oven for 25 minutes. You'll know they're done when the insides are nice and tender.

While the eggplants are in the oven, use a sharp knife to cut the tortilla wraps into triangles and place them on a baking sheet.

Lightly drizzle the triangles with olive oil and sprinkle with 1 tsp. of cumin and 3 tsp. of sea salt. Place in the oven to back for 20 minutes until they are browned and crispy.

Remove the eggplants from the oven and scoop the insides out completely with a large spoon. You should just have the skins left.

Put the lemon juice, 2 T of olive oil, 0.25 tsp. of salt, and 0.5 tsp. of cumin into a food processor and add the eggplant flesh. Pulse until the ingredients are a well-combined textured mixture.

Drizzle with a tad of olive oil and serve with the crispy cumin tortilla chips!

# Salad

Salads are a great healthy addition to any meal, but sometimes they fall flat. Amp up the flavor with this chapter of salad recipes for a fresh alkalizing boost that will introduce you to a whole new world of salad making. Ditch the boring romaine and ranch and try out these recipes that are sure to impress!

# Double "A" Quinoa Salad

This salad is an explosion of apples and almonds on a satisfying bed of quinoa. Try out this recipe for a perfect combination of sweet and salty all in one healthy dish.

Total Prep and Cooking Time: 25 min.

Difficulty Level: Intermediate

Yields: 4 Servings

## Ingredients:

Quinoa - 0.5 c

Granny Smith apple - 1 c chopped

Water - 1 c

Dried cranberries - 0.25 c

Almonds - 0.25 c sliced

Lemon juice - 1.5 tsp.

Spinach - 3 c

Sunflower seeds - 2 T

Raspberry vinaigrette - 0.5 c

**Instructions:**

Measure out your quinoa and rinse it in the sink to remove the grain's bitter coating.

Place a small pot on medium heat with the water and quinoa combined. Follow the quinoa's package instructions for correct cooking times.

Start another pan on medium heat to toast the almonds and sunflower seeds. Add the nuts to the dry pan (no oil!) and toast for about one minute until they are golden brown and crispy.

Start chopping your apple. it is up to you if you want the fruit peeled or not.

In a medium bowl, toss the chopped apple pieces with the lemon juice to keep them fresh.

When the quinoa is done the cooking, remove the pot from the heat and place in the fridge to cool completely. Do not mix the salad when the quinoa is hot because it will wilt the other fresh ingredients.

Once the quinoa is cooled, toss it together with the chopped apple, spinach, and dried cranberries.

Drizzle your desired amount of dressing over the top and mix to distribute evenly. Top your delicious bowl with the toasted nuts and seeds. Serve and enjoy!

# Rainbow Super Salad

Produce from every color of the rainbow adorns this salad. It is a deliciously fresh boost of energy to get through your busy day.

Total Prep and Cooking Time: 30 min.
Difficulty Level: Intermediate
Yields: 4 Servings

**Ingredients:**
Baby kale - 4 c
Watermelon- 1 c
Cucumber - 1 c sliced
Avocado - 1 sliced
Raspberries - 0.5 c
Papaya - 1 c
Baby broccoli - 1 c
Toasted almonds - 0.5 c
Goji berries - 0.25 c
Olive oil - 0.5 c
Sea salt - 1 pinch
Dates - 4 whole

Master tonic (recipe below) - 0.5 c

Fresh ginger - 0.25 c chopped

Turmeric - 2 knobs chopped

Horseradish - 2 T minced

Onion - 0.5 c chopped

Lemon juice - 0.5 c

Organic apple cider vinegar - 32 oz.

Jalapeno pepper - 0.5 c chopped

Garlic - 0.25 c minced

**Instructions:**

Master tonic must be made two weeks ahead of time for its immune-boosting effect. Add all tonic ingredients to a mason jar containing the apple cider vinegar and shake until evenly mixed.

Let your tonic set for about two weeks and shake occasionally to maintain even distribution.

After the tonic has set, strain out all the ingredients and transfer the vinegar mixture to a bottle or jar for safekeeping.

Mix the olive oil and your master tonic together in a medium bowl, adding a pinch of salt as you mix.

Blend together the goji berries and dates until you have a smooth mixture and add it to the olive oil tonic mix.

Toss all the remaining ingredients together to make the salad and top with toasted almond slices.

Drizzle desired amount of dressing over your rainbow creation and enjoy!

## Shredded Golden Beet Salad

For an unconventional healthy pick-me-up, try this shredded golden beet salad. The veggies are all shredded and coated in a creamy herb and garlic dressing for a scrumptious easy bite.

Total Prep and Cooking Time: 20 min.

Difficulty Level: Intermediate

Yields: 4 Servings

## Ingredients:

Baby kale - 4 c cut into strips

Carrots - 2 shredded

Yellow bell pepper - 1 large shredded

Golden beet - 4 large shredded

Green onions - 4 large sliced

Dressing - 1 c

Basil - 1 tsp.

Oregano - 1 tsp.

Tamari - 1 T

Tahini - 3 T

Apple cider vinegar - 2 oz.

Olive oil - 2 oz.

Ginger - 1-inch chunk minced

Garlic - 3 cloves minced

**Instructions:**

Add all of your dressing ingredients into a blender and pulse until the mixture is smooth and slightly creamy.

Make sure to place it in the refrigerator to chill for an hour before serving on top of the salad.

Shred your beets, peppers, and carrots with a kitchen grater into a large bowl so that you have small minced-like strips.

Add the sliced kale and onions to your bowl of other shredded veggies.

Mix all the veggies together so that they are evenly distributed

Drizzle the salad with your dressing and serve!

Bright Brunch Salad

Salad accompanies almost any meal. Why should brunch be any exception? Try this recipe for a sweet salad that is the perfect substitution for unhealthy sugary brunch foods.

Total Prep and Cooking Time: 20 min.

Difficulty Level: Easy

Yields: 6-8 Servings

**Ingredients:**

Blackberries - 1 c

Strawberries - 1 c

Mandarin orange - 1 c

Mixed greens - 2 bags

Lime juice - 0.25 c

Stevia - 1 T

Dijon mustard - 2 T

Olive oil - 0.25 c

Salt - 0.5 tsp.

Black pepper - 0.25 tsp.

Goat cheese - 0.5 c

Pecans - 0.5 c chopped

**Instructions:**

In a small bowl, whisk together the lime juice, stevia, mustard, salt, pepper, and olive oil until they are well combined.

In a separate bowl, toss together the fruit and mixed greens.

Drizzle with your desired amount of dressing.

Sprinkle on goat cheese and pecans for the final touch.

Serve and enjoy!

# Grilled Zucchini Salad

Fire up the grill for this deliciously light but filling salad. Stuffed with greens and topped with a spicy mint dressing, this recipe is sure to be a summer favorite!

Total Prep and Cooking Time: 20 min.

Difficulty Level: Interme

Yields: 6 Servings

## Ingredients:

Watercress - 2 c

Zucchini - 6 large

Sea salt - 0.25 tsp.

Chili-mint dressing - 0.5 c

Fresh mint leaves - 0.5 c

Red chili - 1 pepper minced

Lemon juice - 1 T

Lemon zest - 1 tsp.

Olive oil - 6 T

Sea salt - 0.25 tsp.

Pepper - 0.25 tsp.

**Instructions:**

Slice your zucchinis lengthways into long flat slices and sprinkle them with sea salt while you preheat your grill.

Lay the slices of zucchini on the grill, closing the lid and cooking for 4 minutes on each side. You should be able to see dark grill marks.

While your zucchini is cooking, make your chili-mint dressing by adding all of the dressing ingredients to a food processor or blender and pulsing until the mixture is smooth.

Spread the watercress on a dish and top with the grilled zucchini.

Drizzle the salad with your chili-mint dressing and serve!

## Dragon Fruit Salad

Ditch the boring lunch routine with this unique dragon fruit salad. Dragon fruit looks exotic, but it is actually sold in most grocery stores so you can try this quick and yummy salad with ease.

Total Prep and Cooking Time: 15 min.
Difficulty Level: Easy
Yields: 2 Servings

**Ingredients:**
Avocado - 1 large sliced
Raw macadamia nuts - 0.5 c
Pomegranate seeds - 0.5 c
Dragon fruit - 1 large diced
Fresh greens - 4 c
Dressing - 1 c
Lemon juice- 0.25 c
Lime juice - 1 T
Lime zest - 1 tsp.
Olive oil - 0.25 c
Agave - 2 tsp.

Avocado - 0.5 large

Water - 2 T

Sea salt - 0.25 tsp.

Mint - 5 leaves

## Instructions:

Add all of the dressing ingredients to a blender or food processor and pulse until the mixture is creamy and smooth.

Divide your greens of choice into two large bowls and top with the sliced avocado, macadamia nuts, pomegranate seeds, and diced dragon fruit.

Drizzle with your creamy lime and mint dressing and serve!

## Mexican Quinoa Salad

Take a bite of the south with this Mexican quinoa salad that combines fresh ingredients with bold flavors. It is a must-try for Mexican food lovers!

Total Prep and Cooking Time: 20 min.

Difficulty Level: Easy

Yields: 6-8 Servings

**Ingredients:**

Avocado - 1 c diced

Red bell pepper - 1 c finely diced

Adzuki beans - 1 can

Quinoa - 1 c

Water - 2 c

Coconut oil - 6 T

Cumin - 1 tsp.

Cilantro - 3 T chopped

Scallions - 1 bunch sliced

Lime juice - 6 T

Salt and pepper - To Taste

**Instructions:**

Place a saucepan over low heat with the quinoa, salt, and water.

Cover the pan and simmer for about 15-20 minutes until the water is fully absorbed.

Remove from the heat and set aside.

Whisk together the olive oil, cumin, and lime juice in a small bowl. Add some salt and pepper to your taste.

In a large bowl, fold together the avocado, bell pepper, beans, quinoa, and scallions until they are evenly mixed.

Drizzle your desired amount of dressing over the salad and stir.

Serve your salad warm or set aside to chill and enjoy later.

# Roasted Beet Bowl with Lentils

This salad recipe is the perfect unique dish to add to any meal. Earthy flavors from the beets work harmoniously with the garlic and herbs to create a hearty artisan salad.

Total Prep and Cooking Time: 55 min.
Difficulty Level: Easy
Yields: 4 Servings

## Ingredients:

Asparagus - 2 bunches chopped

Beets - 8 medium

Water - 4 c

Olive oil - 4 tsp.

Garlic - 2 cloves

Cilantro - 1 c

Avocado - 2 large

Lentils - 2 c

Almond milk - 4 T

Salt and pepper - To Taste

Also needed: baking sheet

**Instructions:**

Preheat your oven to 425 degrees.

Wash your lentils thoroughly and place a pot over medium heat.

Fill the pot with the lentils and water and cook for about 15 minutes until the water has been absorbed.

Meanwhile, wash your beets thoroughly and then peel them.

Spread your beats out on a greased baking sheet and place in the preheated oven for 45 minutes.

Coat your asparagus completely with the olive oil to add to the baking sheet for the last 10 minutes remaining of the beets' cooking time.

Blend lime juice, salt and pepper, cilantro, avocado, and garlic until smooth. Add the almond milk and blend until you have a smooth sauce.

In a large bowl, mix together the lentils, asparagus, and beets until evenly combined.

Drizzle your salad with your avocado sauce. Mix and serve.

# Lunch

Lunch can be a stressful undertaking for those with a busy schedule. It is all too easy to pop out to a fast-food restaurant on your lunch break rather than pack ahead, but most restaurants are full of acidic foods lying in wait to ruin your diet, not to mention they do quite a number on your wallet. This chapter offers the solution to maintaining your diet with a busy schedule. These recipes are easy to make and full of flavor to save your wallet and healthy habits!

# Avocado Chickpea Salad Wraps

Chicken salad wraps make room for this hearty nutritional option. Try these avocado chickpea wraps for a hand-held lunch that will boost your energy for the rest of the day!

Total Prep and Cooking Time: 20 min.

Difficulty Level: Easy

Yields: 3 Servings

## Ingredients:

Tomato - 1 c sliced

Red onion - 0.5 c

Lemon juice - 2 T

Cilantro - 0.25 c

Chickpeas - 1.5 c

Avocado - 1 c

Sea Salt - 1 tsp.

Gluten-free wrap - 3 wraps

**Instructions:**

Rinse the chickpeas and throw them in a large bowl with your avocado. Smash the chickpeas and avocado with a fork or potato masher.

Add your salt, lemon juice, onion, cilantro, and mix thoroughly.

Spread a few spoonfuls of your chickpea mixture each wrap and add tomato slices.

Serve and enjoy.

## Garlic Roasted Mushroom Bowl

This hearty grain bowl is full of garlicky goodness and earthy mushrooms for a satisfying lunch with that home-cooked feel. Try this recipe for a healthy meal that will stick to your bones and please your taste buds.

Total Prep and Cooking Time: 35 min.

Difficulty Level: Intermediate

Yields: 6 Servings

**Ingredients:**

Olive oil - 2 T

Water - 2 c

Crimini baby Bella mushrooms - 16 oz.

Uncooked quinoa -  1 c

Garlic - 4 cloves minced

Shallot - 0.25 c minced

Goat cheese - 0.5 c

Sliced almonds - 0.5 c

Salt and pepper - To Taste

Also needed: baking sheet

**Instructions:**

Preheat your oven to 425 degrees and rinse your quinoa under cool water.

Place a medium pot over high heat with the quinoa and water and bring the mixture to a boil.

Once bubbling, reduce the heat to low and simmer for 15 minutes until the water is absorbed. Remove from heat but keep the pot covered.

While you cook your quinoa, rinse your mushrooms and slice them into halves.

Place the slices on a baking sheet and drizzle with olive oil. Sprinkle on salt and pepper to your preference.

Place the baking sheet of mushrooms into the oven and roast for 10 minutes.

Remove the mushrooms from the oven and add the chopped garlic and shallots to the slices. Continue to cook for another 10 minutes.

Use a fork to fluff your quinoa and transfer into a bowl.

Add a spoonful of mushrooms on top and sprinkle with the goat cheese and almonds.

Serve and enjoy!

## Pesto Power Bowl

Easy to make, full of energy-boosting ingredients, and delicious flavors...this lunch bowl has it all! Try this for a recipe filled with greens that you actually want to eat!

Total Prep and Cooking Time: 10 min.
Difficulty Level: Easy
Yields: 2 Servings

**Ingredients:**

Avocado - 1 sliced

Quinoa - 1 c

Chia seeds - 1 T

Hemp seeds - 2 T

Homemade pesto - 0.25 c

Garlic - 1 clove

Pine nuts - 0.25 c

Kale - 1 c

Basil - 2 c

Lemon juice - 1 tsp.

Olive oil - 4 T

Salt and pepper - To Taste

**Instructions:**

Wash your quinoa under cool water and cook to manufacturer's instructions.

Add your homemade pesto ingredients into a food processor and blend until your mixture is smooth.

Divide your quinoa into two bowls and top each with half of the avocado and half of the pesto.

Sprinkle your yummy quinoa bowls with both types of seeds and serve.

# Not Your Average Tomato Soup

A bowl of easy tomato soup is a perfect addition to any chilly autumn day. This unique recipe is prepared so that your veggies are kept raw for that extra alkaline boost without sacrificing flavor.

Total Prep and Cooking Time: 10 min.

Difficulty Level: Easy

Yields: 2 Servings

## Ingredients:

Tomatoes - 10 large

Onion - 1 large chopped

Sweet red peppers - 2 large

Garlic - 2 cloves chopped

Vegetable stock - 0.5 c

Salt and pepper - To Taste

## Instructions:

Pour half of your stock into a medium pan and place on high heat.

Once your stock is boiling, toss in your garlic and onions to steam for about 2 minutes until they are soft.

Pour the rest of your vegetable stock into a blender and add the tomatoes and peppers. Take your steamed onions and garlic and pour that mixture into the blender as well.

Pulse until you're the mixture is smooth and creamy. It should be a thick soup consistency.

Sprinkle on your desired amount of salt and pepper and serve!

## Flavors of Fall Quinoa Bowl

For a bite full of autumn flavors, try this quinoa bowl. Roasted fall veggies are tossed with hearty beans and quinoa for a rustic filling lunch.

Total Prep and Cooking Time: 30 min.

Difficulty Level: Easy

Yields: 4 Servings

### Ingredients:

Carrot - 1 large grated

Beet - 1 large grated

Sweet potato - 1 large grated

Shallots - 2 chopped

Garlic - 4 cloves cooked

Water - 3 c

Quinoa - 2 c

White beans - 15 oz.

Sage - 0.5 sliced

Almond slivers - 0.5 c

Olive oil - 0.25 c

Lemon juice - 1 tsp.

Lemon zest - 1 tsp.

Salt and pepper - To Taste

## Instructions:

Wash and drain your quinoa while you put a pot on medium heat. Add in the quinoa, garlic, water, and shallots. Cook for 20 minutes. You will know it is done when the liquid is absorbed.

Stir in the rest of the ingredients and add your desired amount of salt and pepper.

Serve and enjoy!

# Avocado Lettuce Wraps

Lunch can't get any fresher than this! These hand-held lettuce wraps are stuffed with flavorful veggies for an easy-to-go meal.

Total Prep and Cooking Time: 10 min.

Difficulty Level: Easy

Yields: 2 Servings

## Ingredients:

Red onion - 0.5 c diced

Cilantro - 2 T

Avocado - 1 large sliced

Tomato - 1 c diced

Butter lettuce leaf - 2 leaves

Jalapeno pepper - 2 T

Cumin - 0.5 tsp.

Salt and pepper - To Taste

## Instructions:

Spread the avocado on each butter lettuce leaf.

Stack all your fixings by adding onion, cilantro, tomato, salt, a sprinkle of cumin, and pepper.

Fold the lettuce leaf in half for an easy on-the-go wrap.

## Spicy Summer Avocado Soup

Just because the weather is warm doesn't mean you can't enjoy a bowl of soup! This fresh summer avocado soup packs a spicy punch and is served chilled.

Total Prep and Cooking Time: 10 min.
Difficulty Level: Easy
Yields: 2 Servings

### Ingredients:

Tomatoes - 7 large chopped

Olive oil - 2 T

Vegetable stock - 1 c

Red chili pepper - 1 medium chopped

Avocado - 1 large

Spinach - 2 c

Cucumbers - 1.5 large chopped

Lemon juice - 2 T

Fresh ginger - 1.5" chunk chopped

Salt and pepper - To Taste

**Instructions:**

Put all the ingredients in a blender. Pulse until mixture is smooth and creamy. It should be thick, but if the consistency is too heavy for your taste, just add more vegetable stock and blend.

This soup can be served chilled or slightly warmed over the stove. It should never be boiled!

**Mango Curry Bowl**

This tropical tasting bowl contains almost every color of the rainbow paired perfectly with a yummy coconut and mango curry sauce. it is creamy, fresh, and delicious!

Total Prep and Cooking Time: 45 min.

Difficulty Level: Intermediate

Yields: 2 Servings

**Ingredients:**

Broccoli florets - 1 c

Green beans - 1 c

Lentils - 0.5 c

Water - 1 c

Purple cabbage - 1 c shredded

Onion - 3 T diced

Sweet potato - 1 c diced

Cauliflower florets - 4 c

Coconut oil 1 tsp.

Cashew halves - 2 T

Sesame seeds - 0.5 tsp.

Parsley - 1 tsp. minced

Cilantro - 1 tsp. mixed

Coconut mango sauce - 0.5 c

Curry powder - 1 tsp.

Turmeric - 0.25 tsp.

Mango - 1 large diced

Coconut milk - 0.5 c


Also needed: baking sheet


**Instructions:**

While you line a baking sheet with parchment, preheat your oven to 400 degrees.

Mix the diced sweet potato cubes with the coconut oil and half of the curry powder until all the pieces are evenly covered.

Spread the sweet potato bits across the baking sheet and put it in the oven for 25 minutes. Occasionally reach in there and mix the pieces up to ensure even cooking.

While your potato pieces are cooking, make your coconut mango dressing by throwing all the sauce ingredients in a blender and pulsing until the mixture is creamy and smooth. Pour it into a jar and set it aside until later.

Put a pan over medium heat with coconut oil and toss in the onion and the other half of the curry powder.

Let the onions brown for one minute before adding the water and lentils and letting the mixture come to a boil.

Reduce the lentil mixture to a simmer and cover with a lid to cook for 15 minutes. You can make sure the lentils are done by checking to see if all the liquid was absorbed.

Fold in the parsley and cilantro and take the mixture off the heat.

Put a pot with water on the stove on high heat and lightly boil your greens until they are brightly colored. They should cook for about 2-3 minutes.

Use a food processor to pulverize the cauliflower florets to make cauliflower rice. The texture should be mealy and grainy.

Scoop a generous portion of cauliflower rice into your bowls and top with the steamed broccoli, green beans, shredded cabbage, lentils, and roasted sweet potato.

Drizzle the bowls with your coconut mango sauce and top it with sesame seeds and cashews to serve.

# Dinner

A common misconception about healthy eating is that it can't be filling. Not true! This chapter is full of filling, hearty dinner recipes that will give your body a nutritious boost. They are full of flavor and many of them play off of some of your traditional dinner favorites. Take a step towards healthy living without sacrificing the fun of food!

# Spicy Sweet Potato Mexican Skillet

Try this spinoff of a Mexican skillet stuffed to the brim with spicy sweet potatoes and tempeh. it is fresh, yummy, and full of protein to fill your belly alkaline style.

Total Prep and Cooking Time: 25 min.
Difficulty Level: Intermediate
Yields: 4 Servings

**Ingredients:**
Tempeh - 1 block
Coconut oil - 4 T
Red pepper - 1 large
Onion - 1 large
Jalapeno pepper - 1 large
Avocado - 1 large
Garlic - 2 cloves
Lime juice - 2 T
Chili powder - 0.25 tsp.
Sweet potato - 1 large diced
Taco seasoning - 1 T
Cilantro - 2 T minced

Salt and pepper - To Taste

## Instructions:

Place a large pan on medium heat with 2 T of coconut oil.
Toss in your sweet potatoes and cook them for 4 minutes
covered to soften them. Remove the cover and cook for 3
more minutes to crisp up and brown the outsides.

Heat the rest of the coconut oil in a second skillet on
medium heat.

Add the onions to the skillet and cook until they are soft. At
this point, toss in the garlic, jalapeno, and red pepper and
continue to cook until these are also softened and slightly
browned.

Use a kitchen grater to shred the tempeh block into the
skillet with all the vegetables. This will make the tempeh
resemble ground beef.

Sprinkle on the chili powder, salt, and taco seasoning and
stir until everything is evenly combined.

When the tempeh begins to brown, drain the grease from
the pan and gently fold in the sweet potatoes.

Top your skillet with lime juice, cilantro, and sliced
avocado and serve!

## Coconut Vegetable Curry over Quinoa

This light and creamy curry are easy to make but sure to impress. Follow the recipe or add in your favorite veggies to make a dish unique to your palette.

Total Prep and Cooking Time: 30 min.
Difficulty Level: Intermediate
Yields: 4 Servings

**Ingredients:**
Water - 2.5 c
Onion - 1 chopped
Garlic - 2 cloves minced
Coconut milk - 2 c
Green peas - 1 c
Zucchini - 4 c cubed
Quinoa - 1 c
Curry powder - 2 T
Sea salt - 0.5 tsp.

**Instructions:**

Place a saucepan over high heat and add in 2 c of water and the quinoa. Sprinkle with the salt and bring to a boil.

Once the quinoa boils, turn down the heat so that the mixture is set at a simmer and cook for 20 minutes until the liquid has been absorbed.

In a second saucepan, bring the coconut milk to a boil and then turn down to medium heat.

Toss your garlic and onion into the coconut milk and cook while occasionally stirring for a few minutes.

Pour in the curry powder and let the mixture cook for 2 more minutes.

Add the remaining water and zucchini to the mixture and simmer it for about 15 minutes before adding the peas and a sprinkle of salt.

Give the mixture a good long stir to make sure everything is incorporated and then remove from the heat and pour over the quinoa.

Serve and enjoy!

## Vegetable Lo Mein

An alkaline diet doesn't have to mean missing out. Swap the Chinese takeout with this vegetable lo mein recipe for a delicious dish that isn't lacking in flavor or nutrients.

Total Prep and Cooking Time: 30 min.
Difficulty Level: Intermediate
Yields: 4 Servings

### Ingredients:

Onion - 1 large

Mushrooms - 1 c sliced

Red pepper - 1 large

Green pepper - 1 large

Fresh ginger - 1 T

Toasted sesame oil - 1 T

Sesame seeds - 1 T

Grapeseed oil - 2 T

Agave - 1 T

Red pepper flakes - 1 tsp.

Onion powder - 1 tsp.

Sea salt - 0.5 tsp.

Spelt spaghetti noodles - 1 box

Lime juice - 1 T

**Instructions:**

Cook your spelt spaghetti noodles according to the manufacturer's instructions.

Place a pan on medium heat with the grapeseed oil and cook the peppers and onions until they are softened for about 5 minutes.

Add in the mushrooms and ginger to cook for another 3-4 minutes until they are also softened.

Pour your sesame oil, and agave over the cooking veggies and sprinkle on your red pepper flakes, onion powder, and sea salt. Stir so that everything is evenly incorporated.

Take the pan off of the heat and fold in your spelt spaghetti noodles making to mix everything well.

Top with sesame seeds and a drizzle of lime juice and serve!

# Crispy Flatbread Pizza

Pizza is one of the most famous cheat meals, probably because it is so delicious. Try this recipe to curb those greasy pizza cravings without having to cheat on your healthy habits.

Total Prep and Cooking Time: 55 min.
Difficulty Level: Hard
Yields: 6 Servings

## Ingredients:

Green pepper - 1 large sliced

Onion - 0.5 large sliced

Mushrooms - 1 c sliced

Brazil nut cheese - 0.5 c

Sauce - 1 c

Onion - 2 T chopped

Roma tomatoes - 5 large

Agave - 2 T

Oregano - 1 tsp.

Onion powder - 1 tsp.

Sea salt - 1 tsp.

Basil - 1 tsp.

Grapeseed oil - 2 T

Dough

Water - 1 c

Grapeseed oil - 2 T

Agave - 2 T

Sea salt - 1 tsp.

Oregano - 1 tsp.

Onion powder - 1 tsp.

Sesame seeds - 2 T

Spelt flour - 1.5 c

Also needed: baking sheet

**Instructions:**

Preheat your oven to 400 degrees while you coat a baking sheet in grape seed oil

Add all of your dry dough ingredients to a large bowl and pour in half of the water gradually until you can form the mixture into a dough ball.

Spread your dough out onto the baking sheet and brush it lightly with grapeseed oil. Use a fork to poke scattered holes in the dough.

Place the baking sheet in your oven and bake for 12-15 minutes until the crust is just barely golden brown.

While your crust is baking, start on the tomato sauce. Remove the skins from the tomatoes by using a sharp knife to make small "x" cuts on both ends of each tomato. Place them in boiling water for one minute.

Quickly transfer the tomatoes into an ice bath for 30 seconds to shock them. The skin should now easily slide off.

Put your tomatoes and all the other sauce ingredients in a blender or food processor and pulse until the mixture is smooth. (If you love chunky sauce, just under-blend the mixture a tad).

When the crust is looking lightly toasted, pull it out of the oven and spread it with a generous heap of your tomato sauce.

Sprinkle the pizza with your veggies of choice (mushrooms, green peppers, and onions are a great combo) and top with brazil nut cheese.

Bake your pizza for another 15 minutes until the crust is golden brown and the nut cheese is spread and melted.

Cut into slices and serve!

**Sprout Stir-Fry**

This stir-fry is packed with veggies and doesn't sacrifice flavor. Try this recipe for a nutritious stir-fry dish doused in a sauce that will convert the most avid soy sauce fans to this healthier alkaline option.

Total Prep and Cooking Time: 45 min.

Difficulty Level: Intermediate

Yields: 4 Servings

**Ingredients:**

Green pepper - 1 large sliced

Celery - 1 stalk chopped

Brussel sprouts - 8 sprouts halved

Broccoli - 1 bunch chopped

Onion - 1 large

Ginger - 2 tsp. minced

Kale - 0.5 c ribboned

Mung bean sprouts - 1 c

Coconut oil - 2 T

Garlic - 2 cloves minced

Water - 3 c

Quinoa - 1.5 c

Gluten-free tamari - 0.5 c

## Instructions:

Put a pot with the water and quinoa on high heat and bring it to a boil. When it reaches a boil, add one clove of minced garlic and turn the heat down to low to let the mixture simmer.

Cover and cook for 20 minutes until the liquid has been completely absorbed.

In a separate pan, simmer the other half of the minced garlic, tamari, and one tsp. of ginger on medium heat until you have a thick syrupy sauce.

While the quinoa and sauce are in the works, heat a large wok with coconut oil. Add the rest of the ginger and onions to the wok and cook them until they are slightly browned. Add the rest of your vegetables minus the sprouts to the wok and mix them thoroughly. Cover with a lid for the veggies to steam for about 7 minutes until they are slightly softened but still have a bit of a bite.

Remove the vegetables from the heat and fold in the sauce so that everything is coated.

Fill a bowl with first a large scoop of quinoa and then a scoop of vegetables. Top with the sprouts and serve!

## Fajita Skillet

Busy days happen. Suddenly it is dinner time and you do not have anything planned to make. Try this fajita recipe for a quick and easy, one-pan meal ready in just 15 minutes.

Total Prep and Cooking Time: 15 min.
Difficulty Level: Easy
Yields: 6 Servings

**Ingredients:**

Spelt flour tortillas - 12 small
Green pepper - 0.5 c sliced
Red pepper - 0.5 c sliced
Mushrooms - 3 c sliced
Onions - 1.5 c sliced
Cayenne - 0.5 tsp.
Oregano - 2 tsp.
Basil - 2 tsp.
Onion powder - 2 tsp.
Sea salt - 2 tsp.
Lime juice - 1 T

Grapeseed oil - 1 T

**Instructions:**

Put a large skillet on the medium-high heat with your grapeseed oil.

Toss in your vegetables cut into long slices and sprinkle them with all your herbs and seasoning.

Mix the ingredients well and then cook for 5 minutes until the veggies get soft and slightly browned.

Serve on the spelt tortillas (try warming them for 10 seconds in the microwave first) and top with fresh tomato salsa and lime juice.

# Zoodles and Lentil Meatballs

Swap out carb-heavy traditional pasta and meatballs for this zoodles and lentil meatballs recipe. it is filling and delicious, and most importantly it won't weigh you down with a bunch of acidic carbs.

Total Prep and Cooking Time: 55 min.

Difficulty Level: Intermediate

Yields: 6 Servings

## Ingredients:

Old-fashioned oats - 0.5 c

Egg - 1 large

Carrots - 1 c shredded

Onion - 0.5 c diced

Vegetable broth - 1.5 c

Dried lentils - 0.75 c

Oregano - 1 tsp.

Tomato paste - 1.5 T

Garlic - 2 cloves minced

Parsley - 0.25 c chopped

Salt - 0.25 tsp.

Pepper - 0.25 tsp.

Prepared zoodles - 5 c


Also needed: baking sheet


**Instructions:**

Rinse your lentils under cold water and allow them to drain.

Place a pot over medium heat with the broth and add the drained lentils. Bring the mixture to a high simmer before dropping the temperature to medium-low and cooking for 25 minutes. There should always be a bit of water over the lentils to assure they do not dry out.

While your lentils are cooking, start a second pan on medium-low heat with the olive oil. Sizzle your onions for about 5 minutes until they are soft and a little browned.

Toss in your carrots to cook for 2 additional minutes before adding the garlic. Stir for one more minute until everything is combined.

Pour the oats and parsley into a blender or food processor and pulse until the oats are broken up. Add your lentils and your onion mixture as well as oregano, salt, tomato paste, and pepper.

Pulse a couple of times until the mixture seems combined before adding the egg that acts as a glue for the meatballs. Continue to blend until all the ingredients are combined and the mixture has a mealy texture.

Rest your meatball mixture in the fridge for ten minutes while you heat your oven to 425 degrees and grease a baking sheet.

Roll your meatball mixture into balls about 1 inch wide and lay them in rows on your baking sheet.

Cook in the oven for 10 minutes. Pull out your meatballs to turn them and then cook for another 10 minutes until the outsides are browned and firm.

Serve over prepared zoodles with red tomato sauce.

# Turmeric Chickpea Burgers

Have a cook-out alkaline style with these chickpea burgers. They pack a bold punch with turmeric and cayenne flavors and are great for dinner any time of the year.

Total Prep and Cooking Time: 20 min.
Difficulty Level: Intermediate
Yields: 4 Servings

**Ingredients:**

Chickpeas - 1 can

Garlic - 2 cloves

Onion - 1 small

Chickpea flour - 4 T

Cayenne pepper - 0.5 tsp.

Turmeric powder - 1 tsp.

Grapeseed oil - 1 T

Sea salt - 1 tsp.

Parsley - 0.25 c

Pepper - 0.5 tsp.

**Instructions:**

Pour the grapeseed oil in a large pan on medium heat and toss in the onions and garlic. Cook for 5 minutes until they are soft and slightly browned and then remove from heat to cool.

Grind up the canned chickpeas in a food processor until it has a mealy texture. Make sure to scrape down the sides to catch any chickpea chunks hiding.

Toss in your onions, garlic, cayenne, turmeric, salt, and pepper and pulse until they are evenly combined with the chickpeas. Fold in the parsley last.

Sprinkle chickpea flour onto a flat plate and scoop a small golf ball-sized amount of chickpea mixture into your hands. Press the ball down unto the plate to form a patty coated with chickpea flour. Flip the patty to coat the other side so there is a light coating of flour on all sides of the patty.

Put your large pan back on medium heat and add more grapeseed oil. When the oil is hot, place your chickpea patties in the pan and cook each side for 3 minutes until the edges are crispy and browned.

Serve your patties with a salad or lettuce wraps and enjoy!

## Spicy Garlic Risotto

This recipe is proof that diets can be delicious. Try it out for a creamy cauliflower risotto with a whole lot of flavor. Beware the chili garlic sauce; it will have you licking your plate and begging for more!

Total Prep and Cooking Time: 30 min.
Difficulty Level: Intermediate
Yields: 4 Servings

## Ingredients:

Coconut milk - 0.5 c
Red bell peppers - 2 T diced
Onion - 0.5 c chopped
Cauliflower - 14 oz.
Banana pepper - 1 pepper sliced
Basil - 1 bunch chopped
Lime juice - 0.5 T
Pumpkin seeds - 0.25 c crushed toasted
Chili garlic sauce - 1 c
Gluten-free Tamari - 2 tsp.
Agave - 1 T

Chili paste - 2 T

Red pepper flakes - 1 tsp.

Ginger - 0.5 T grated

Almond milk - 0.5 c

Avocado - 1 small

Garlic - 3 tsp. minced

**Instructions:**

Make your dressing by pouring all of the chili garlic sauce ingredients into a blender and pulsing until you have a smooth mixture. If you want to thin the sauce a bit, just add 1 or 2 T of water and blend.

Take your cauliflower head and chop off all the leaves and stems.

Pulverize the cauliflower by pulsing it in a food processor. You want the consistency to be similar to rice.

Place a pan on medium heat with coconut oil and toss in your garlic and onions to cook for 2 minutes until lightly browned.

Add your red peppers and cauliflower rice to the mixture and continue to cook for another 3 minutes.

Pour in your almond milk and continue to cook on medium as you stir. Make sure all the cauliflower rice is coated.

Remove the pan from the heat and add the lime juice.

Sprinkle in salt and pepper to taste and mix up the risotto.

Transfer your risotto to a bowl and add green peppers, chili peppers, and the basil.

Top with the crushed nuts and a drizzle of garlic sauce.

(You can also top your risotto with tofu for extra protein).

# Dessert

Just because you choose to live healthy doesn't mean that you have to give up dessert! This chapter is full of delicious dessert recipes to satisfy any sweet tooth. They are easy to make so you aren't tempted to grab an overly-sugar snack, and they are based on some of your cheat-day favorites. Stay on track without losing the sweet side of life!

# Guilt-free Apple Crumble

As fall approaches, the desserts close in. do not miss out on your favorite fall flavors and try this recipe for apple crumble that won't knock you off track.

Total Prep and Cooking Time: 20 min.

Difficulty Level: Easy

Yields: 4 Servings

## Ingredients:

Gluten-free rolled oats - 0.5 c

Green apple - 2 c sliced

Pear - 2 c sliced

Nutmeg - 1 tsp.

Cinnamon - 2 tsp.

Raw almonds - 0.5 c chopped

Coconut oil - 1 T

Stevia - 1 tsp.

## Instructions:

Place a pan over medium heat with the coconut oil.

Toss in the sliced pears, apples, cinnamon, and nutmeg.
Cook for about 5 minutes while occasionally stirring until
the fruit is soft and tender.

In a small bowl, mix together the almonds, oats, stevia, and
a little extra cinnamon.

Distribute the fruit mixture evenly into four bowls.

Top your fruit compote with the sweet oats mixture and
serve!

## Strawberry "Ice Cream"

There's nothing better than a scoop of ice cream on a hot summer day. Make your own with this easy strawberry "ice cream" recipe that is dairy-free and alkaline friendly.

Total Prep and Cooking Time: 20 min.

Difficulty Level: Intermediate

Yields: 4 Servings

## Ingredients:

Strawberries - 0.5 c

Coconut milk - 1 c

Bananas - 2 frozen

Hemp seeds - 1 T

Goji berries - 1 T

Unsweetened coconut flakes - 2 T

Chia seeds - 1 T

Ice - 2 c

**Instructions:**

Combine the ice, strawberries, chia seeds, coconut milk, and bananas in a blender and puree until creamy and smooth.

Add the goji berries and fold them into the mixture until evenly spread throughout.

Pour the mixture into a baking tray and smooth with a spatula to make sure it is even.

Sprinkle the hemp seeds and coconut flakes over the top and place in the freezer overnight. The "ice cream" is ready when the mixture is firm to the touch.

Scoop out the desired amount of dessert with a spoon and serve!

# Chocolate Chip Scones

Choosing to live alkaline isn't as difficult as it seems, especially when it comes to baked goods. Try out this recipe for a warm chocolate chip scone that melts in your mouth and makes your tummy smile.

Total Prep and Cooking Time: 20 min.

Difficulty Level: Intermediate

Yields: 4 Servings

## Ingredients:

Light coconut milk - 1 c

Frozen coconut oil - 0.5 c grated

Baking powder - 2.5 tsp.

Stevia - 0.25 c

Salt 0.5 tsp.

Vanilla extract - 1 tsp.

Chickpea flour - 2 c

Cacao nibs - 0.5 c

Also needed: baking sheet

**Instructions:**

While you line a baking sheet with parchment, preheat your oven to 350 degrees.

Whisk together your stevia, flour, salt, and baking powder until they are evenly mixed.

Add your grated frozen coconut oil to the bowl of dry ingredients and use a form to mash the frozen oil until it combines with the dry mixture to form a grainy dough.

Gradually pour in the vanilla extract and coconut milk into your dough-in-process. Be gentle as you stir the wet ingredients into the dry ones because you do not want to overwork your dough. It should be thick and a bit sticky to the touch.

Fold in the cacao nibs.

Shape the dough into a large mounding circle on your baking sheet and cut it, using a sharp knife, into 8 equally sized slices.

Bake your scone dough for 20 minutes before removing to quickly re-cut the 8 slices and separate them slightly.

Sprinkle a pinch of stevia over the tops of the pieces to give them a crunchy sweet coating.

Return the scones to the oven for 5 more minutes until the pastries are golden.

Cool for 5-10 minutes before serving warm or storing for up to 3 days.

## Very Berry Funnel Cake

Take a trip to the fair with these berry funnel cakes! They are fresh, sweet, and most importantly not covered in grease.

Total Prep and Cooking Time: 20 min.
Difficulty Level: Intermediate
Yields: 2 Servings

### Ingredients:

Garbanzo bean flour - 2 c

Spelt flour - 1 c

Coconut milk - 1 c

Agave - 8 T

Mixed berries - 1 c

Stevia - 1 T

Grapeseed oil - 0.5 c

### Instructions:

Mix the funnel cake batter by combining the flour, coconut milk, and agave and stir until the batter is thick and smooth.

Put a pan over medium heat and fill up to about one inch with the grapeseed oil. There should be enough oil to completely cover one cake.

Fill a disposable plastic bag (cake decorating bags work best) with the cake batter and cut a small hole in the corner.

Once the oil is bubbling, begin to squeeze your batter into the pan in squiggle-like movements to create the shape of a funnel cake.

Leave the cake to cook in the oil for 5 minutes until it is golden brown. No need to flip it.

Remove the funnel cake and let it cool and drain on a paper towel.

Toss your mixed berries with the stevia while your funnel cake cools a bit.

Top your cooled funnel cake with a scoop of mixed berries and serve.

# No-Bake Cacao Pistachio Balls

For a quick bite that will satisfy your sweet tooth, try these cacao pistachio balls. They have the texture and chocolatey flavor of a brownie with a crunchy nutty coating!

Total Prep and Cooking Time: 10 min.

Difficulty Level: Easy

Yields: 12 Servings

## Ingredients:

Almonds - 0.25 c

Pistachios - 0.5 c

Cacao powder - 0.5 c

Shredded unsweetened coconut - 0.5 c

Coconut oil - 0.5 c

Almond meal - 1 c

Chia seeds - 1 T

Dates - 4 large

**Instructions:**

Fill a medium bowl with hot water and soak the almonds and dates for one hour to soften them. Make sure to remove the seeds from the dates!

Toss your softened dates and almonds into a blender or food processor with the shredded coconut, cacao powder, coconut oil, chia seeds, and half of the pistachios. Pulse until you have a mealy texture.

Move your mixture to a large bowl to rest for a few minutes until the chia seeds break down and expand.

Crush up the rest of your pistachios. For a finer chop, use a food processor.

Roll the dough mixture into small balls and then roll them in the crushed pistachio for a fully covered coating.

Serve or save in the fridge for up to a week!

**Extra Chocolatey Banana Bread**

Calling all chocolate lovers! This banana bread is a must-try for those who love everything chocolate. Try it out for a moist slice to satisfy your sweet tooth!

Total Prep and Cooking Time: 60 min.

Difficulty Level: Intermediate

Yields: 10 Servings/1 Loaf

**Ingredients:**

Cacao nibs - 1 c

Coconut flour - 0.5 c

Cocoa powder - 0.5 c

Baking powder - 1 tsp.

Baking soda - 1 tsp.

Vanilla extract - 1 tsp.

Coconut oil - 0.25 c

Almond butter - 0.5 c

Eggs - 4 large

Sea salt - 0.25 tsp.

Bananas - 2.5 c mashed

Also needed: 9x5" loaf pan

## Instructions:

Preheat your oven to 350 degrees while greasing your loaf pan to prevent sticking.

Mix together the bananas, nut butter, vanilla extract, coconut oil, and eggs in a large bowl until the ingredients are all evenly combined.

Add in the sea salt, baking powder, baking soda, coconut flour, and cocoa powder into the bowl and mix until you have a smooth thick batter.

Fold in the cacao nibs evenly throughout the batter.

Pour your batter into the greased loaf pan, spreading it evenly with a spatula.

Place the pan into the preheated oven and bake for one hour. Insert a toothpick into the center and make sure it comes out clean to ensure the loaf is cooked all the way through.

Remove the loaf of banana bread from the pan and place on a rack to cool before serving.

# Baked Strawberry Blender Doughnuts

Dough-"not" becomes dough-"yes" with this recipe for baked strawberry doughnuts. The best part? You can easily make them in your blender!

Total Prep and Cooking Time: 35 min.
Difficulty Level: Intermediate
Yields: 8 Servings

## Ingredients:

Egg whites - 1 c

Banana - 1 c mashed

Baking powder - 1.5 tsp.

Gluten-free multi-purpose flour - 1.75 c

Light coconut cream - 0.5 c

Strawberries - 1 c

Salt - 0.25 tsp.

Stevia - 0.5 c

Vanilla - 1 tsp.

Glaze - 1 c

Stevia - 0.5 c

Strawberries - 0.5 c

Non-dairy coconut Greek yogurt - 0.5 c

Also needed: doughnut baking tray

**Instructions:**
Grease your donut baking pan while you preheat the oven to 350 degrees.

Mix together your flour, baking powder, salt, and stevia in a large bowl.

Blend the strawberries, banana, and egg whites with your coconut cream until the mixture is smooth.

Add in your dry ingredients in small portions at a time to avoid pockets of dryness in the batter.

Once blended smoothly, add in your vanilla extract and give a couple of extra pulses to mix thoroughly.

Pour your batter carefully into the donut holes of your baking sheet. Be careful to not overspill or the shapes will be off.

Bake for 15-20 minutes until the dough is a golden brown.

While you wait for the batter to bake, combine all the ingredients for the glaze in a blender and mix until the liquid-smooth.

Once your doughnuts are golden brown, you can remove them from the oven. Remove the treats from the pan and set them aside to cool.

Brush the glaze over you doughnuts making sure all the sides are covered and serve!

## Raw Lemon Balls

A sour-sweet treat ready in only 10 minutes for a quick but impressive last-minute dessert.

Total Prep and Cooking Time: 10 min.

Difficulty Level: Easy

Yields: 6 Servings

### Ingredients:

Lemon juice - 0.5 c (or 3 lemons)

Agave - 1.5 T

Coconut flour - 0.25 c

Almond flour - 1.5 c

Himalayan salt - 0.5 tsp.

Coconut oil - 0.25 c

Vanilla extract - 2 tsp.

Shredded unsweetened coconut flakes - 0.5 c

### Instructions:

Fill a small bowl with the unsweetened coconut flakes.

Add all of the other ingredients to a food processor or blender and pulse until you have a well-combined mealy dough.

Spoon out a bit of dough at a time and use your palms to roll the small spoonful into balls.

Roll the lemon balls in the coconut flakes until the outside layer is completely covered.

Firm for 5-10 minutes in the refrigerator and serve.

# Smoothies and Drinks

Every day we are surrounded by so many sugary drinks that it is easy to slip up. Swap your morning coffee or cheat-day milkshake with any one of these deliciously sweet smoothies. They all contain raw fruit for that alkalizing effect and combine nutrients to give you an energizing boost. Whether you're a decadent chunky monkey fan or like to steer towards the tropical fruits, there's something for you in this chapter!

**Red Velvet Protein Booster**

This smoothie tastes just like a slice of red velvet cake and will provide you with an extra energy boost to get you through the day.

Total Prep and Cooking Time: 10 min.
Difficulty Level: Easy
Yields: 1 Serving

**Ingredients:**

Cucumber - 1 medium

Beet - 1 medium

Almond butter - 1 T

Almond milk - 1 c

Chocolate Alkamind Protein Powder - 1 scoop

**Instructions:**

Blend the raw beet until it is thoroughly shredded.

Add all the rest of your ingredients.

Blend until smooth and creamy.

Serve and enjoy!

# Sweet Green Smoothie

Get your daily dose of greens in a deliciously sweet smoothie. Try this recipe for a nutritious snack that hides your greens behind yummy sweet flavors.

Total Prep and Cooking Time: 10 min.

Difficulty Level: Easy

Yields: 1 Serving

## Ingredients:

Banana - 1 large

Green apple - 1 large peeled

Kiwi - 1 large

English cucumber - 0.5 c sliced

Mint - 12 leaves

Spinach - 1 c

Lemon juice - 1 T

Lemon zest - 1 tsp.

Stevia - 1 tsp.

Coconut oil - 1 T

Water - 0.25 c

**Instructions:**

Add all your ingredients to a blender and puree until creamy and smooth.

Pour into your favorite glass and enjoy!

# Chocolate Covered Frozen Banana Smoothie

This recipe tastes like a chocolate-covered banana in c. Try it out for an energy boost that will satisfy your sweet tooth.

Total Prep and Cooking Time: 10 min.

Difficulty Level: Easy

Yields: 2 Servings

**Ingredients:**

Coconut milk - 2 c

Bananas - 2 frozen

Chia seeds - 2 T

Cacao nibs - 2 T

Cacao powder - 2 T

Coconut oil - 2 T

**Instructions:**

Add all your ingredients except the chia seeds to a blender and puree until creamy and smooth.

Toss in the chia seeds and pulse once or twice to evenly distribute them.

Pour into your favorite glass and enjoy!

# PB&J Smoothie

This smoothie will bring up memories of your childhood with every sip. Try this recipe for peanut butter and a jelly flavored smoothie with hidden greens for an extra boost of nutrients.

Total Prep and Cooking Time: 10 min.
Difficulty Level: Easy
Yields: 2 Servings

## Ingredients:

Banana - 1 frozen

Strawberries or mixed berries - 1 c frozen

Almond milk - 2 c

Raw almond butter - 4 T

Spinach - 2 c

## Instructions:

Add the spinach and almond milk to your blender and puree until the mixture is smooth.
Toss in all your other ingredients and blend until creamy and smooth.

Pour into your favorite glass and enjoy!

# Snickerdoodle Smoothie

Touches of cinnamon make this creamy smoothie taste just like a snickerdoodle. Enjoy hidden greens masked by delicious sweet spices instead of reaching for those cookies and keep your healthy eating habits on track.

Total Prep and Cooking Time: 10 min.

Difficulty Level: Easy

Yields: 2 Servings

**Ingredients:**

Almond milk - 1 c

Avocado - 1

Banana - 2 frozen

Spinach - 1 c

Cinnamon - 2 tsp.

Vanilla extract - 1 T

**Instructions:**

Add all the ingredients to your blender and blend until the mixture is smooth.

Pour into your favorite glass and enjoy!

# Tropical Turmeric Smoothie

For a taste of island living, try this tropical-flavored smoothie! It is packed with raw fruits and veggies to give your body an alkalizing boost!

Total Prep and Cooking Time: 10 min.

Difficulty Level: Easy

Yields: 2 Servings

## Ingredients:

Almond milk - 0.5 c

Ginger - 1 tsp.

Mango - 1 large diced

Banana - 1 large frozen

Water - 1.25 c

Carrots - 4 peeled and chopped

Lemon juice - 1 T

Turmeric powder - 0.25 tsp.

## Instructions:

Add all the ingredients to your blender and blend until the mixture is smooth.

Pour into your favorite glass and enjoy!

## Carrot Cake Smoothie

Skip the slice of cake and try this carrot cake smoothie instead. It is cool and refreshing with all the sweetness of a slice of cake!

Total Prep and Cooking Time: 10 min.

Difficulty Level: Easy

Yields: 2 Servings

### Ingredients:

Coconut milk - 1 c

Vanilla extract - 0.5 tsp.

Nutmeg - 0.25 tsp.

Cinnamon - 0.25 tsp.

Ginger - 0.25 tsp.

Old-fashioned oats - 1 c cooked

Banana - 1 c frozen

Carrot - 0.5 c grated

### Instructions:

Add all the ingredients to your blender and blend until the mixture is smooth.

Pour into your favorite glass and enjoy!

# Watermelon Spritzer

This recipe is perfect for a hot summer's day. The sweetness of the watermelon mixed with the sour lime makes for an easy refreshing spritz without all the sugar.

Total Prep and Cooking Time: 10 min.

Difficulty Level: Easy

Yields: 2 Servings

## Ingredients:

Sparkling water - 0.25 c

Lime zest - 1 tsp.

Lime juice - 1 T

Watermelon - 4 c

## Instructions:

Add all the ingredients to your blender and blend until the mixture is smooth.

Pour into your favorite glass and enjoy!

## Skittle Smoothie

Strawberries and sour lemons swirl together in this cool refreshing mashup. For a little taste of the rainbow in an easy, healthy drink, try this skittle flavored smoothie!

Total Prep and Cooking Time: 10 min.

Difficulty Level: Easy

Yields: 2 Servings

## Ingredients:

Lemon juice - 0.5 c

Lime juice - 1 T

Lime zest - 1 tsp.

Non-dairy yogurt - 1 c

Strawberries - 1 c

## Instructions:

Add all the ingredients to your blender and blend until the mixture is smooth.

Pour into your favorite glass and enjoy!

## Strawberry Steamer

For a romantic Valentine's Day drink or just anytime you need a warm, pink pick-me-up, try this strawberry almond steamer beverage! It is super easy to make and will warm you to the core with a smile on your face.

Total Prep and Cooking Time: 10 min.
Difficulty Level: Easy
Yields: 2 Servings

### Ingredients:

Almond extract - 0.8 tsp.

Vanilla extract - 0.5 tsp.

Coconut manna - 3 T

Strawberries - 10 large

Almond milk - 2 c

Coconut nectar - 1 tsp.

Liquid stevia - 10 drops

### Instructions:

Put a small pot on medium-low heat and slowly warm up your almond milk until it is just barely hot to the touch.

Pour the warmed almond milk into a blender and toss in the rest of your ingredients. Pulse until the mixture is smooth and a little bit frothy.

Pour into your favorite mug and enjoy!

# A Lime in the Coconut

Put the lime in the coconut and mix it all up! Try this refreshing smoothie for a healthy dose of the tropics wherever you are.

Total Prep and Cooking Time: 10 min.
Difficulty Level: Easy
Yields: 2 Servings

## Ingredients:

Almond milk - 1 c

Lime juice - 1 T

Lime zest - 1 tsp.

Unsweetened coconut flakes - 0.5 c

Coconut flesh - 0.5 c

Bananas - 2 frozen

## Instructions:

Add all the ingredients to your blender and blend until the mixture is smooth.

Pour into your favorite glass and enjoy!

## Matcha Monster

Matcha has taken the world by storm, and it is no surprise. The green tea flavor of Matcha pairs perfectly with almost anything to create an antioxidant-rich, metabolism-boosting drink!
In this recipe, the sweetness of the banana pairs perfectly with the Matcha for a sweet refreshing smoothie.

Total Prep and Cooking Time: 10 min.
Difficulty Level: Easy
Yields: 2 Servings

**Ingredients:**
Matcha powder - 2 tsp.
Almond milk - 1 c
Spinach - 1 c
Banana - 1 frozen

**Instructions:**
Add all the ingredients to your blender and blend until the mixture is smooth.
Pour into your favorite glass and enjoy!

# Snacks

Snacking. Otherwise known as the diet killer. When those afternoon munchies hit, it is hard not to reach into the cabinet for whatever you have on hand. However, that usually means something acidic or unhealthy. This chapter is full of easy snack recipes that you can make ahead to enjoy when those cravings start creeping up. Try one of them out for a midday energy boost that will make your taste buds sing!

# Mini Veggie Fritters

Curb your cravings for crispy fried food with these mini veggie fritters. They are perfect hand-held snacks with an alkalizing veggie twist!

Total Prep and Cooking Time: 30 min.
Difficulty Level: Intermediate
Yields: 10 Servings

**Ingredients:**
Red pepper - 0.75 c chopped
Red onion - 0.25 c chopped
Corn - 0.75 c
Parsley - 2 T chopped
Garlic - 1 clove minced
Paprika - 0.25 tsp.
Cayenne pepper - 0.5 tsp.
Cumin - 1 tsp.
Water - 0.5 c
Garbanzo bean flour - 0.75 c
Coconut oil - 2 T

**Instructions:**

Add all of your dry ingredients to a medium bowl and mix them together.

Whisk in your water until the batter is smooth and clumps.

Fold in your chopped vegetables, mixing until they are distributed evenly throughout the batter.

Put a pan on medium-high heat with the coconut oil and heat until the oil is sizzling.

Use a spoon to drop palm-sized circles of batter into the pan. Fill the pan with as many fritters as possible for each batch.

Cook for about 5 minutes until the fritter is browned and stiff enough to lift easily.

Flip each one and repeat the step above.

Remove your fritters from the pan and place on a rack or paper towel to cool and drain.

Serve and enjoy!

## Peanut Butter Bars

Whip up these baked peanut butter bars for an energy-rich snack that's easy to take on the go. They are sweet, nutty bites that will keep you going during long busy days.

Total Prep and Cooking Time: 35 min.

Difficulty Level: Intermediate

Yields: 12 Servings

### Ingredients:

Almond butter - 0.75 c

Oats - 1 c

Garbanzo bean flour - 0.75 c

Almond milk - 0.5 c

Vanilla extract - 1 T

Stevia - 0.5 c

Baking soda - 1 tsp.

Salt - 0.25 tsp.

Also needed: 8x8" baking dish

**Instructions:**

Line your baking dish with parchment while heating the oven to 350 degrees.

Use an electric mixer to whip together the almond butter and the stevia until it is a fluffy mixture.

Continue to mix on low speed while adding in the flour, baking soda, vanilla extract, and oats.

Pour in the almond milk gradually until the mixture develops a doughy consistency.

Pull the dough out of the mixing bowl and press it into the center of the baking dish. Make sure the surface is even.

Place the dish in the oven and bake for 20 minutes until the surface is firm and the top is golden colored.

Put the dish aside to cool and use a knife to slice the bars into 12 squares.

Serve or save for up to 1 week.

## Salty Kale Chips

Potato chips move aside for these salty kale chips. This recipe is great for salty snack lovers who have trouble keeping their hands out of the chip bag. They are easy to make and a great healthy substitute for traditional potato chips!

Total Prep and Cooking Time: 20 min.
Difficulty Level: Easy
Yields: 2 Servings

### Ingredients:

Paprika - 1 tsp.
Olive oil - 2 T
Curly kale - 1 bunch
Salt - 1 tsp.

Also needed: baking sheet

### Instructions:

While you remove large kale stems from your bunch, preheat your oven to 300 degrees.

Tear the kale into bite-sized pieces and dry extremely well with a paper towel.

In a bowl, combine the kale pieces with paprika, olive oil, and salt. Mix well so that all of the greens are coated.

Pour your kale onto a baking tray and spread the leaves out evenly so that they are all evenly cooked.

Cook for 15 minutes until the leaves look extra crispy and slightly browned. Keep a careful watch while they are cooking because it is very easy to overcook and turn ashy if you have a strong oven.

Serve in a bowl for a guilt-free salty snack!

Protein-Packed Sweet Potato Cookies

For a midday energy boost, try these sweet potato cookies. They are sweet and filled with autumn spices, but most importantly they are packed with protein to keep you healthy, happy, and energized!

Total Prep and Cooking Time: 20 min.

Difficulty Level: Intermediate

Yields: 8-12 Servings

## Ingredients:

Almond butter - 0.5 c

Oat flour - 0.25 c

Eggs whites- 2 large

Cooked sweet potato - 0.75 c mashed

Baking soda - 1 tsp.

Cinnamon - 1 tsp.

Vanilla extract - 1 tsp.

Maple syrup - 2 T

Pepitas - 2 T

Chia seeds - 2 T

Craisins - 0.25 c


Also needed: baking sheet


## Instructions:

Start preheating your oven to 375 degrees while you line a cookie sheet with parchment.

Add the sweet potato, egg whites, and almond butter to a large bowl and whisk together until smooth.

Pour the cinnamon, seeds, vanilla, syrup, and craisins into the batter and fold throughout the mixture.

Add your baking soda and oat flour gradually as you stir.

Mix together until it resembles a doughy consistency.

Scoop morsels of cookie dough onto the baking sheet. You should have enough dough to make 8-10 cookies depending on the desired size

Bake for 10 minutes until the edges of the cookies become browned. Remove from the oven and cool off on a baking sheet before enjoying.

## Healthier Hummus Dip

Traditional hummus is already a great healthy snack, but this recipe adds in hidden vegetables with a bite of dill. This dip is great for those who want to go the extra mile in their alkaline diet.

Total Prep and Cooking Time: 10 min.
Difficulty Level: Easy
Yields: 6-8 Servings

### Ingredients:
Avocado - 1 large
Chickpeas - 1 c
Ground sesame seeds - 2 T
Dill - 0.25 c

### Instructions:
Add all of your ingredients to a food processor and pulse until your mixture is creamy in texture.
Scoop into a bowl and serve with a side of your favorite veggies!

# Pumpkin To-Go Bars

As fall rolls around, so does everything pumpkin spice. Unfortunately, most of these autumn flavored eats threaten to throw you off your alkaline eating habits. Try these pumpkin to-go bars when you're craving fall spices. This recipe is perfect for pumpkin spice addicts!

Total Prep and Cooking Time: 30 min.
Difficulty Level: Easy
Yields: 4 Servings

**Ingredients:**

Coconut oil - 1 T

Raw almonds - 0.25 c chopped

Hemp seeds - 1 T

Chia seeds 0 2 T

Cinnamon - 1 tsp.

Vanilla extract - 1 tsp.

Unsweetened shredded coconut flakes - 0.25 c

Fresh pumpkin (or organic pumpkin puree) - 1 c

Gluten-free oats - 2 c

Also needed: 8x8" baking dish

**Instructions:**

Grease your baking pan with coconut oil while preheating your oven to 350 degrees.

Combine all your ingredients into a medium bowl and mix well so that everything is evenly distributed.

Scoop the gooey mixture into an even layer in your greased pan.

Back for 20 minutes. When the bars are done the top will be firm and golden brown.

Remove from the oven to cool for 10 minutes.

Slice into evenly sized bars and serve or store in an airtight container for as long as four days.

## **Salty and Sweet Potato Chips**

These alkalizing potato chips are the perfect combination of salty and sweet for midday snack cravings. The recipe substitutes traditional potatoes for sweet potatoes to give you a crispy salty snack that won't throw you off track.

Total Prep and Cooking Time: 90 min.

Difficulty Level: Intermediate

Yields: 4 Servings

### **Ingredients:**

Coconut oil - 2 T

Sweet potatoes - 4 large

Sea salt and pepper - To Taste

Also needed: mandolin, baking sheet

### **Instructions:**

Preheat your oven to 200 degrees.

Thinly slice your sweet potatoes using a mandolin. You can slice them with a knife but they will be thicker and not bake as well.

Toss your sliced potatoes into a large bowl and toss with the coconut oil until they are evenly coated. Sprinkle on salt and pepper and mix thoroughly.

Line your baking sheet with parchment and spread the potato slices out on it evenly.

Place the baking sheet into the oven for 45 minutes.

Pull your potatoes out of the oven and flip them. Bake for an additional 45 minutes to 1 hour until the slices look fairly toasted.

Cool on the baking sheet to allow the chips to crisp up. Add a sprinkle of salt or pepper to taste and serve.

# Roasted Rosemary Almonds

This recipe yields delicious bite-sized munchies for an energizing afternoon snack. Try these salty rosemary almonds to curb your hunger during the day or put them out at a party as an appetizer for guests to munch on. Either way, they promise to be a hit!

Total Prep and Cooking Time: 20 min.

Difficulty Level: Easy

Yields: 2 Servings

## Ingredients:

Olive oil - 2 T

Rosemary - 2 T chopped

Almonds - 1 c

Salt and pepper - To Taste

Also needed: baking sheet

## Instructions:

While you preheat your oven 350 degrees, lightly grease a baking sheet.

Toss the almonds in a bowl containing the olive oil and rosemary until the nuts are well coated.

Toast in the oven for about 15 minutes until the almonds are browned and crispy.

Sprinkle with salt and pepper to taste and serve with an extra sprinkle of rosemary.

# Conclusion

Congratulations! You are now ready to start your journey to healthy living. Taking up the alkaline diet is a big step towards a healthy you, and hopefully, you will enjoy your journey as much as we do and decide to adopt healthy practices into your life for good.

You learned the basic tenets of the alkaline diet like what foods to enjoy guilt-free and what foods to pass on, and you now have the knowledge to start a healthy dict on the right foot with our recipe for the perfect successful cleanse. Continue your natural living plan into the world of medicine by utilizing your new knowledge of herbal medicine.

Take the information you learned and apply it to your life with determination and, most importantly, fun. A diet should not mean sacrifice which is why this book of recipes exists for you to reference and use over again. Don't hesitate to experiment and try new things!

The alkaline diet is a safe and easy way to lose weight and keep it off. As you now know, there is no pesky fasting and no grumbling stomach. You can still enjoy food while keeping your body in the best shape possible. Not only is it a weight-loss tool, but following this diet plan also prevents diseases and ailments that can plague a tired body. You now have a plethora of knowledge in your belt on what foods to eat and what foods to avoid as well as over 50 recipes to try.

**Happy cooking!**